211234
2600K   25

Dynamic Nurse Management

Cabashon Publishing
A Division of Health Educational International, Inc.
San Diego, California

Dynamic Nurse Management

Mark B. Silber, Ph.D.
Janet L. Marlborough, MBA, RN
Eileen M. McLachlan, Ph.D., RN

Continuing Education Instructions

The multiple-choice continuing education (CE) exams that follow are designed to test your understanding of the information provided in *Dynamic Nurse Management*. Five exams are presented as follows:

Exam I covers information provided in Chapters 1 and 2,
Exam II covers information provided in Chapters 3 and 4,
Exam III covers information provided in Chapters 5 and 6,
Exam IV covers information provided in Chapters 7 and 8, and
Exam V covers information provided in Chapter 9.

Each exam is worth 2.0 hours of CE credit (0.2 CEUs) for a total of 10.0 hours of credit (1.0 CEU).

You may submit as many exams as you choose; however, all exams that you select to complete should be submitted at one time.

Before starting the CE program, be sure to review the learning objectives for each exam you elect to complete. Then read the chapter(s) that correspond to the exam, focusing on key points related to the learning objectives. After reading the chapter(s), take the corresponding exam(s). There is only one correct answer for each question. You may photocopy the answer form at the end of the examination booklet and submit your answers on the photocopied form.

To receive CE credit, complete the enrollment information on the following page and submit it along with your completed answer form and enrollment fee to Health Education International, Inc. (HEI).

Upon receipt of all your completed exams, HEI will score them and return the results and correct answers to you. A passing score is required for CE credit. (The passing score varies from test to test, but it is never less than 70%). Your CE certificate will be issued within 30 days after you submit your answers.

Illegible or incompleted forms may delay scoring and return of your CE certificate and test results.

If you have any questions, please write or call:

Health Education International, Inc.
11770 Bernardo Plaza Court, Suite 308
San Diego, CA 92128
(619) 451-0342

Enrollment Information

PLEASE PRINT CLEARLY

Check one: ☐ RN   ☐ LVN   ☐ Other (please specify)_________________

____

Name ____

Address ____

City ______________________________ State _____ Zip ____________

Phone (_____) ____

Social Security No. _________________ Current Position _____________

License number(s) and State(s) of licensure _______________________

____

I have enclosed __________ ($10 per exam or $40 if all five exams are submitted.)

☐ I have enclosed an additional $10.00 for addresses in foreign countries.

☐ My check or money order payable to Health Education International, Inc. is enclosed. (US currency only. Do not send cash.)

☐ Bill my MasterCard®/Visa® (Circle one).

Card No. _____________________________ Expires _______________

Signature____

Exam I — Chapters 1 and 2

Chapter I - Today's Challenges: Goals in Transition
Chapter II - The Changing Hospital

CE Credit: 2.0 Contact hours
Passing Score: 71 % (10 correct answers)

Learning Objectives

1. Recognize recent changes in health care delivery.
2. Explain how changes in health care delivery have affected the nursing profession.
3. Recognize new methods used to control health care costs and increase revenues.
4. Discuss the factors that influence the climate and culture of a hospital.

Exam Questions

1. What has had the biggest impact on health care delivery in recent years?
   a. Technologic advances
   b. Shortage of nurses
   c. Higher patient acuity
   d. Economic pressures

2. The goal of health care has changed from one of eliminating disease to one of
   a. decreasing patient charges.
   b. promoting well-being.
   c. consolidating resources.
   d. providing safe patient care.

3. The Medicare program reimburses for hospitalization by charging
   a. a fee for service.
   b. per capita charges.
   c. amounts based on groups of diagnoses.
   d. rates similar to those charged by preferred-provider and health maintenance organizations (PPOs and HMOs).

4. After years of growth and high profits, hospitals are now faced with cost containment, aggressive marketing strategies, and
   a. supply and demand of the marketplace.
   b. the high cost of staff made up entirely of registered nurses (RNs).
   c. increase in available services.
   d. development of high-cost technology.

5. As a result of financial constraints in health care delivery, nurses now must balance patient-care cost with
   a. appropriate staffing numbers.
   b. adequate resources.
   c. quality patient care.
   d. patient-care demands.

6. Traditionally, the priority goal in nursing has been "mission" rather than
   a. self-care.
   b. management.
   c. strategy.
   d. productivity.

7. To deal effectively with the crises in health care today, the nurse-manager must have a realistic perception of the challenges, adequate situational support, and
   a. financial security.
   b. appropriate staffing resources.
   c. effective management skills.
   d. a degree in business management.

8. You are the chief executive officer of a large corporation. Because of the rising employee health care costs, you are likely to
   a. stop providing medical benefits.
   b. join a PPO.
   c. continue current health benefits.
   d. increase the operating budget.

9. For a hospital to be profitable, patients' length of stay must be decreased, productivity increased, and the number of patients served
   a. increased.
   b. kept at a break-even point.
   c. decreased.
   d. restructured.

10. The ratio of cost to charge must be analyzed for each department of a
hospital. The goal is to ensure that charges are
    a. lower than costs.
    b. reduced.
    c. increased.
    d. higher than costs.

11. A positive organizational climate most likely accompanies which type
of management style?
    a. Decentralized
    b. Participative
    c. Contractual
    d. Bureaucratic

12. One of the operational values that contributes to creating a climate of
growth is
    a. production.
    b. care.
    c. investment.
    d. reward.

13. When an effective nurse-manager allows staff members to solve problems and make decisions, the manager is controlling
    a. people.
    b. personal needs.
    c. productivity.
    d. progress.

14. One of the most important skills a nurse can develop is learning how
to
    a. teach.
    b. learn.
    c. create.
    d. survive.

Exam II — Chapters 3 and 4

Chapter 3 - The Effective Nurse - Manager
Chapter 4 - Communication: The Nerve Center of Management

CE Credit: 2.0 Contact hours
Passing Score: 75% (12 correct answers)

Learning Objectives

1. Recognize management skills that result in effective leadership behaviors.
2. Discuss the components of conflict resolution that lead to organizational growth.
3. Describe the process of communication and its importance in nursing management.
4. Describe effective communication skills and strategies.

Exam Questions

1. A nurse-manager who spends time with staff members identifying problems and allowing the members to provide solutions is concerned with
   a. process.
   b. doing things right.
   c. looking good.
   d. people.

2. Primary characteristics of a peak performer are large amounts of energy, singleness of purpose, enjoyment of a challenge, and
   a. collegial support.
   b. knowledge of group dynamics.
   c. excellent interpersonal skills.
   d. a stable personal life.

3. Nurse-managers who are effective negotiators give information in small amounts, ask questions, and make use of
   a. mutual direction.
   b. delay tactics.
   c. local labor laws.
   d. sound advice.

4. Nurse-managers are encouraged to share leadership functions with others; however, only the manager can represent the department to the rest of the hospital and be responsible for staff
   a. performance.
   b. contributions.
   c. education.
   d. behavior.

5. A nursing unit is considering going from 8-hour shifts to 12-hour shifts. Some nurses like the idea, some do not. There are no budgetary constraints. The first step an effective nurse-manager would take would be to
   a. survey staff members for their opinions.
   b. wait and see what happens.
   c. design a research project that measures work effectiveness after 8- and 12-hour shifts.
   d. make a decision based on the success of other units.

6. Nurses at a hospital are requesting changes in the standards of patient care and improved personnel benefits. The nurse-manager should view this action as
   a. something to be fought until the end.
   b. an unavoidable situation.
   c. a positive step for growth and change.
   d. a management failure.

7. Effective conflict resolution encourages communication and centers on
   a. personalities.
   b. problem solving.
   c. compromise.
   d. win-lose strategies.

8. Nurses on the pediatric unit are in major disagreement over the dress code. Half the nurses want to wear scrubs, the other half want to wear printed tops with white pants or skirts. Neither group is willing to change. A professional issues committee is organized to address the problem. This is an example of
   a. redirecting behavior.
   b. reallocating resources.
   c. reframing perspectives of the conflict.
   d. realigning underlying forces.

9. Positive outcomes of effective conflict resolution include problem solving, increased understanding of the issues, and
   a. strategies for negotiation.
   b. goal achievement.
   c. increased influence of the staff nurse.
   d. selective perception.

10. The stages of communication involve message producing, sending, and
    a. retaining.
    b. analyzing.
    c. receiving.
    d. understanding.

11. A medical unit needs more staff because of a higher acuity of patients and increased census. However, the budget request for more staff members was not approved. This most likely is due to the unit manager's lack of
    a. concern for the staff's feelings.
    b. knowledge about the budgeting process.
    c. skill in communicating unit accomplishments and fiscal needs.
    d. ability to define resource allocations.

12. Open communication involving sincere interest in others decreases anxiety and helps create
    a. predictability in relationships.
    b. deeper meanings.
    c. high productivity.
    d. motivation among staff members.

13. The chief of surgery and the nurse-manager of the operating room are arguing about staffing. They finally calm down and agree that their primary goal is quality patient care. They have done which of the following?
    a. Avoided dynamic dialogue
    b. Identified a commonality
    c. Limited the message
    d. Examined the context

14. The flow of information that is horizontal, informal, and primarily concerned with task coordination takes place in which type of organizational structure?
    a. Matrix
    b. Flexible
    c. Formal
    d. Hierarchal

15. To ensure that staff members understand what is happening, an effective nurse-manager will create a democratic environment, improve personal communication techniques, and
    a. increase the flow of vertical messages.
    b. require collaboration.
    c. deal with complexity.
    d. help staff members develop communication skills.

16. A nurse-manager is concerned about the many changes taking place in the hospital and on the unit. The staff members are upset and anxious. The nurse-manager should do which of the following?
    a. Rely on informal communication networks
    b. Wait for upper management to make changes
    c. Schedule staff meetings to share concerns
    d. Start a communication book and encourage everyone to make entries

Exam III — Chapters 5 and 6

Chapter 5 - Managing Motivation
Chapter 6 - Developing Power Strategies

CE Credit: 2.0 Contact hours
Passing Score: 72% (16 correct answers)

Learning Objectives

1. Recognize the factors that influence motivation.
2. Discuss what the nurse manager can do to manage motivation among employees.
3. Recognize various sources of power.
4. Recognize factors associated with the effective use of power.
5. Discuss methods of developing power skills and habits.

Exam Questions

1. Primary influences on motivation in the workplace are specific individual needs and goals and the
   a. social milieu.
   b. economic environment.
   c. organizational tasks and management practices.
   d. authority given the individual.

2. Attractive salaries, opportunities for socialization, and chances for creativity are called
   a. growth needs.
   b. incentives.
   c. motivation factors.
   d. dissatisfaction avoidance needs.

3. Both Maslow and Herzberg agreed that all persons are first motivated by needs based on
   a. physiology and security.
   b. dissatisfiers.
   c. extrinsic fear and reward.
   d. self-actualization.

4. According to Herzberg, it is important to balance the opportunities for psychologic growth and the
   a. process of job enrichment.
   b. social opportunities for self-realization.
   c. influence of task significance.
   d. avoidance of dissatisfiers.

5. Organizational policy, working conditions, supervisors, salary, and security are all examples of
   a. factors that can cause dissatisfaction.
   b. job enrichment motivators.
   c. positive work perceptions.
   d. growth and development needs.

6. A group of staff nurses in an outpatient clinic developed their own job descriptions and designed a clinical ladder program. What kind of activity is this?
   a. The manager's function
   b. A process of job enrichment
   c. An unlikely one because of lack of employee interest
   d. One essential to employee satisfaction

7. Job descriptions must be based on standards that can be measured objectively to appraise
   a. motivation.
   b. employee satisfaction.
   c. job performance.
   d. accountability.

8. A nurse-manager for a surgical intensive care unit has developed job enrichment programs and allowed staff members to make their own work schedules. Some of the nurses are not interested in job challenge and more responsibility. The nurse-manager should handle this situation by doing which of the following?
   a. Counseling the nurses who are not interested
   b. Giving staff members more authority responsibility
   c. Continuing the job enrichment programs
   d. Taking over the scheduling

9. The nurse-manager should know that the motivation process is primarily
    a. self-released.
    b. associated with affiliation needs.
    c. related to worth of the work.
    d. externally applied.

10. Nurses in an emergency department are concerned about giving advice to callers on the telephone. Someone has suggested developing a telephone triage protocol. The nurse-manager should do which of the following?
    a. Hire a consultant to develop the program
    b. Direct nurses not to give telephone advice because of the legal ramifications
    c. Organize a committee of emergency nurses to examine the problem and recommend a course of action
    d. Write the departmental policies and procedures for giving advice over the telephone

11. A manager offered to send two staff members to a quality assurance seminar (all expenses paid) in return for serving on the audit committee. This is use of which kind of power?
    a. Expert
    b. Referent
    c. Legitimate
    d. Reward

12. An employee's performance is below standard, which results in demotion and transfer. What types of power is the manager using?
    a. Coercive and legitimate
    b. Legitimate and referent
    c. Referent and expert
    d. Expert and reward

13. The clinical nurse specialist who works closely with the nurse-manager most likely has what kinds of power?
    a. Coercive and legitimate
    b. Legitimate and reward
    c. Reward and expert
    d. Expert and referent

14. The night shift of a unit had been working short staffed for 2 weeks, and the patient acuity had been high. One night the nurse-manager appeared on the unit with doughnuts and a personal note of thanks for each night nurse. The type of power the manager showed was
    a. expert.
    b. referent.
    c. reward.
    d. legitimate.

15. Nurses who use power effectively are self-confident, energetic, and view power as
    a. responsibility.
    b. domination.
    c. something given to them.
    d. a four-letter word.

16. The best way for a nurse-manager to have a solid power base is to
    a. increase manager influence.
    b. decrease restrictive power.
    c. increase staff responsibility and influence.
    d. ensure reciprocity.

17. A quiet stare, a moment of silence, and "no" without an explanation from a skilled nurse-manager are which of the following?
    a. Unusual
    b. Used frequently
    c. Unacceptable
    d. Effective

18. To make career advancements, the nurse-manager must like power but remember to emphasize
    a. patient-oriented achievement.
    b. staff recognition and involvement.
    c. successful communication.
    d. job satisfaction.

19. To enhance sources of power, every nurse-manager needs visibility, sponsorship, and a
    a. mentor.
    b. distinctive style.
    c. motivated staff.
    d. large amount of energy.

20. A nurse recently has been promoted to manager of a medical- surgical unit. One of the first things the manager should do is to
    a. develop likability.
    b. begin completing the tasks.
    c. delegate authority.
    d. get to know the staff.

21. One of the basic objectives in cultivating a network of colleagues is to
    a. maintain alliances.
    b. promote organizational programs.
    c. give and collect favors.
    d. increase visibility.

22. A warm, open, friendly style might be interpreted as manipulative unless the manager has
    a. integrity.
    b. expert power.
    c. connections.
    d. enabling power.

Exam IV — Chapters 7 and 8

Chapter 7 - The Nurse-Manager as Change Agent
Chapter 8 - Counseling the Problem Employee

CE Credit: 2.0 Contact hours
Passing Score: 71 % (15 correct answers)

Learning Objectives

1. Recognize inherent factors associated with change.
2. Discuss management strategies that will help staff members deal effectively with change.
3. Discuss the process of implementing change.
4. Recognize factors involved in counseling problem employees.
5. Describe appropriate management strategies for dealing with a problem employee.

Exam Questions

1. Nurse-managers and staff members must realize that change is continuous and
    a. unavoidable.
    b. unrecognized.
    c. ignored.
    d. feared.

2. Persons resist change because security is threatened and
    a. management is poor.
    b. stressors are high.
    c. the unknown is feared.
    d. communication is unreliable.

3. Attitudes toward change are affected by trust in management and by
    a. the job itself.
    b. group influence.
    c. personal strengths.
    d. length of employment.

4. Persons are most likely to accept change if initially they have
    a. been informed in simple direct terms.
    b. accepted the reason for change.
    c. received reward for their efforts.
    d. considered all variables.

5. When planning a change, what should the nurse-manager do first?
    a. Establish goals and objectives
    b. Wait until all the problems have been resolved
    c. Communicate the options for change
    d. Ask for suggestions

6. On a unit that will be instituting primary nursing, which of the following should the nurse-manager do first?
    a. Distribute a questionnaire to determine staff knowledge of primary nursing
    b. Communicate the steps necessary for change
    c. Establish a committee to design new primary nursing tools
    d. Invite speakers to explain the advantages of primary nursing

7. When writing a proposal for change, the nurse-manager should do which of the following?
    a. Include the summary and recommendations at the end of the proposal
    b. Expect to get at least half of what was requested
    c. List the steps of instituting the change
    d. Give a thorough explanation of technical facts

8. The first step in planning change is to
    a. determine the readiness for change.
    b. define the change problem.
    c. state the plan of action.
    d. identify the change process.

9. When determining readiness for change, the nurse-manager must ensure that the level of staff satisfaction is
   a. decreased.
   b. maintained.
   c. encouraged.
   d. increased.

10. One common reason for staff members' resistance to change is
    a. perception of the change as criticism.
    b. an uncooperative group leader.
    c. strength of long-time employees.
    d. lack of communication with management.

11. A staff nurse is continually late for work because of child care problems. The appropriate person to speak to this nurse is the
    a. staff coordinator.
    b. employee assistance counselor.
    c. unit manager.
    d. immediate supervisor.

12. An employee has a disagreeable attitude and does not complete the expected work. The nurse-manager should have the employee do which of the following?
    a. Do the job or expect to lose it
    b. Identify the problem
    c. Take some time off
    d. Visit a professional counselor

13. The first thing to remember when counseling a problem employee is to
    a. give accurate advice.
    b. document all activity.
    c. anticipate defensive behavior.
    d. listen objectively.

14. An employee's problem and solution are the responsibility of the
    a. employee's supervisor.
    b. human resource department.
    c. employee.
    d. top executive.

15. One important objective of a counseling session with a problem employee is to initially
    a. allow the employee to express anger and frustration.
    b. identify the employee's problem behaviors.
    c. determine if the employee can be helped.
    d. develop a course of positive action.

16. A staff nurse has had difficulty adjusting to the unit. Frequent errors in judgement have been made and assignments have not been completed. The first two options the nurse-manager should consider are employee counseling and
    a. termination.
    b. transfer.
    c. education.
    d. peer evaluation.

17. When a problem employee is transferred, the action usually is seen as
    a. punishment.
    b. cost-effective use of personnel.
    c. rehabilitation.
    d. passing the problem along to someone else.

18. Terminating an employee may be easier if it is seen as a managerial responsibility and
    a. an inevitable occurrence.
    b. the only answer to a difficult problem.
    c. part of a process.
    d. the best solution for the employee.

19. After receiving a termination notice, an employee angrily confronted the nurse-manager and said, "You have no right to do this because it wasn't my fault." This behavior should be which of the following?
    a. Expected
    b. Squelched
    c. Redirected
    d. Ignored

20. When being verbally attacked by an angry, defensive employee, the
manager initially should do which of the following?
    a. Document all conversation
    b. Listen to the employee in private
    c. Discuss alternative solutions
    d. Analyze the problem from the employee's point of view

21. After a nurse-manager has dealt with a defensive employee and the
confrontation is over, the manager should help the employee do which
of the following?
    a. Find another job
    b. Recall what has happened
    c. Identify reasons for anger
    d. Receive professional counseling

Exam V — Chapter 9

Chapter 9 - The Emerging Patterns of Management

CE Credit: 2.0 Contact hours
Passing Score: 75% (9 correct answers)

Learning Objectives

1. Discuss the changes in hospital organization as society moves from an industrial to an informational age.
2. Recognize the pressures that are changing the methods of health care production.
3. Recognize management patterns necessary to meet the demands of the emerging informational model.

Exam Questions

1. In the industrial society, traditional hospitals are large, hierarchial, and
   a. reciprocal.
   b. centralized.
   c. decentralized.
   d. horizontal.

2. Management values recently have been influenced by behavioral scientists who promote
   a. achievement and recognition.
   b. time and motion.
   c. product and profit.
   d. task and function.

3. Which corporate structure does the informational model of organization use?
   a. Standardized
   b. Vertical
   c. Centralized
   d. Matrix

4. The changes in the physical environment that currently are influenc-
    ing health care are primarily a result of
    a. the team approach.
    b. political influence.
    c. medical technology.
    d. available information.

5. The new informational paradigm places a premium on managing the
    a. development of human resources.
    b. physical environment.
    c. provision of health and wellness information.
    d. economic pressures from society.

6. Emphasis on the team approach and concern for employee education
    and welfare is a result of which pressure affecting the paradigm shift?
    a. Political
    b. Environmental
    c. Social
    d. Moral

7. The nurse-manager in the informational age is one who combines
    persons and ideas to establish strategies and accomplish goals. This is
    known as the
    a. enabling process.
    b. empowerment ability.
    c. paradigm switch.
    d. system of energy exchange.

8. Two interrelated aspects of leadership include the efficient and wise
    exercise of power and the identification of
    a. environmental feedback.
    b. common goals.
    c. expected behaviors.
    d. legitimate functions.

9. The first step that any hospital's management group should take is to
    a. develop goals and objectives.
    b. determine community health needs.
    c. design the organizational chart.
    d. define institutional values.

10. To increase motivation among staff nurses, managers must match patient requirements with
    a. staff achievement and recognition.
    b. resources and availability.
    c. economic incentives.
    d. a pleasant work environment.

11. In the most successful companies, communication is informal and
    a. structured.
    b. along the chain of command.
    c. hierarchial.
    d. across lines.

12. The nurse-manager of tomorrow most likely will use *less* of which type of power?
    a. Reward
    b. Coercive
    c. Expert
    d. Legitimate

<u>   </u>

Answer Sheet *(You may photocopy this form)*

EXAM I — Chapters 1 and 2

1. ☐a	2. ☐a	3. ☐a	4. ☐a	5. ☐a	6. ☐a	7. ☐a	8. ☐a
☐b	☐b	☐b	☐b	☐b	☐b	☐b	☐b
☐c	☐c	☐c	☐c	☐c	☐c	☐c	☐c
☐d	☐d	☐d	☐d	☐d	☐d	☐d	☐d

9. ☐a	10. ☐a	11. ☐a	12. ☐a	13. ☐a	14. ☐a
☐b	☐b	☐b	☐b	☐b	☐b
☐c	☐c	☐c	☐c	☐c	☐c
☐d	☐d	☐d	☐d	☐d	☐d

EXAM II — Chapters 3 and 4

1. ☐a	2. ☐a	3. ☐a	4. ☐a	5. ☐a	6. ☐a	7. ☐a	8. ☐a
☐b	☐b	☐b	☐b	☐b	☐b	☐b	☐b
☐c	☐c	☐c	☐c	☐c	☐c	☐c	☐c
☐d	☐d	☐d	☐d	☐d	☐d	☐d	☐d

9. ☐a	10. ☐a	11. ☐a	12. ☐a	13. ☐a	14. ☐a	15. ☐a	16. ☐a
☐b	☐b	☐b	☐b	☐b	☐b	☐b	☐b
☐c	☐c	☐c	☐c	☐c	☐c	☐c	☐c
☐d	☐d	☐d	☐d	☐d	☐d	☐d	☐d

EXAM III — Chapters 5 and 6

1. ☐a	2. ☐a	3. ☐a	4. ☐a	5. ☐a	6. ☐a	7. ☐a	8. ☐a
☐b	☐b	☐b	☐b	☐b	☐b	☐b	☐b
☐c	☐c	☐c	☐c	☐c	☐c	☐c	☐c
☐d	☐d	☐d	☐d	☐d	☐d	☐d	☐d

9. ☐a	10. ☐a	11. ☐a	12. ☐a	13. ☐a	14. ☐a	15. ☐a	16. ☐a
☐b	☐b	☐b	☐b	☐b	☐b	☐b	☐b
☐c	☐c	☐c	☐c	☐c	☐c	☐c	☐c
☐d	☐d	☐d	☐d	☐d	☐d	☐d	☐d

17. ☐a	18. ☐a	19. ☐a	20. ☐a	21. ☐a	22. ☐a
☐b	☐b	☐b	☐b	☐b	☐b
☐c	☐c	☐c	☐c	☐c	☐c
☐d	☐d	☐d	☐d	☐d	☐d

(Continued on reverse)

EXAM IV — Chapters 7 and 8

1. ☐ a	2. ☐ a	3. ☐ a	4. ☐ a	5. ☐ a	6. ☐ a	7. ☐ a	8. ☐ a
☐ b	☐ b	☐ b	☐ b	☐ b	☐ b	☐ b	☐ b
☐ c	☐ c	☐ c	☐ c	☐ c	☐ c	☐ c	☐ c
☐ d	☐ d	☐ d	☐ d	☐ d	☐ d	☐ d	☐ d

9. ☐ a	10. ☐ a	11. ☐ a	12. ☐ a	13. ☐ a	14. ☐ a	15. ☐ a	16. ☐ a
☐ b	☐ b	☐ b	☐ b	☐ b	☐ b	☐ b	☐ b
☐ c	☐ c	☐ c	☐ c	☐ c	☐ c	☐ c	☐ c
☐ d	☐ d	☐ d	☐ d	☐ d	☐ d	☐ d	☐ d

17. ☐ a	18. ☐ a	19. ☐ a	20. ☐ a	21. ☐ a
☐ b	☐ b	☐ b	☐ b	☐ b
☐ c	☐ c	☐ c	☐ c	☐ c
☐ d	☐ d	☐ d	☐ d	☐ d

EXAM V — Chapter 9

1. ☐ a	2. ☐ a	3. ☐ a	4. ☐ a	5. ☐ a	6. ☐ a	7. ☐ a	8. ☐ a
☐ b	☐ b	☐ b	☐ b	☐ b	☐ b	☐ b	☐ b
☐ c	☐ c	☐ c	☐ c	☐ c	☐ c	☐ c	☐ c
☐ d	☐ d	☐ d	☐ d	☐ d	☐ d	☐ d	☐ d

9. ☐ a	10. ☐ a	11. ☐ a	12. ☐ a
☐ b	☐ b	☐ b	☐ b
☐ c	☐ c	☐ c	☐ c
☐ d	☐ d	☐ d	☐ d

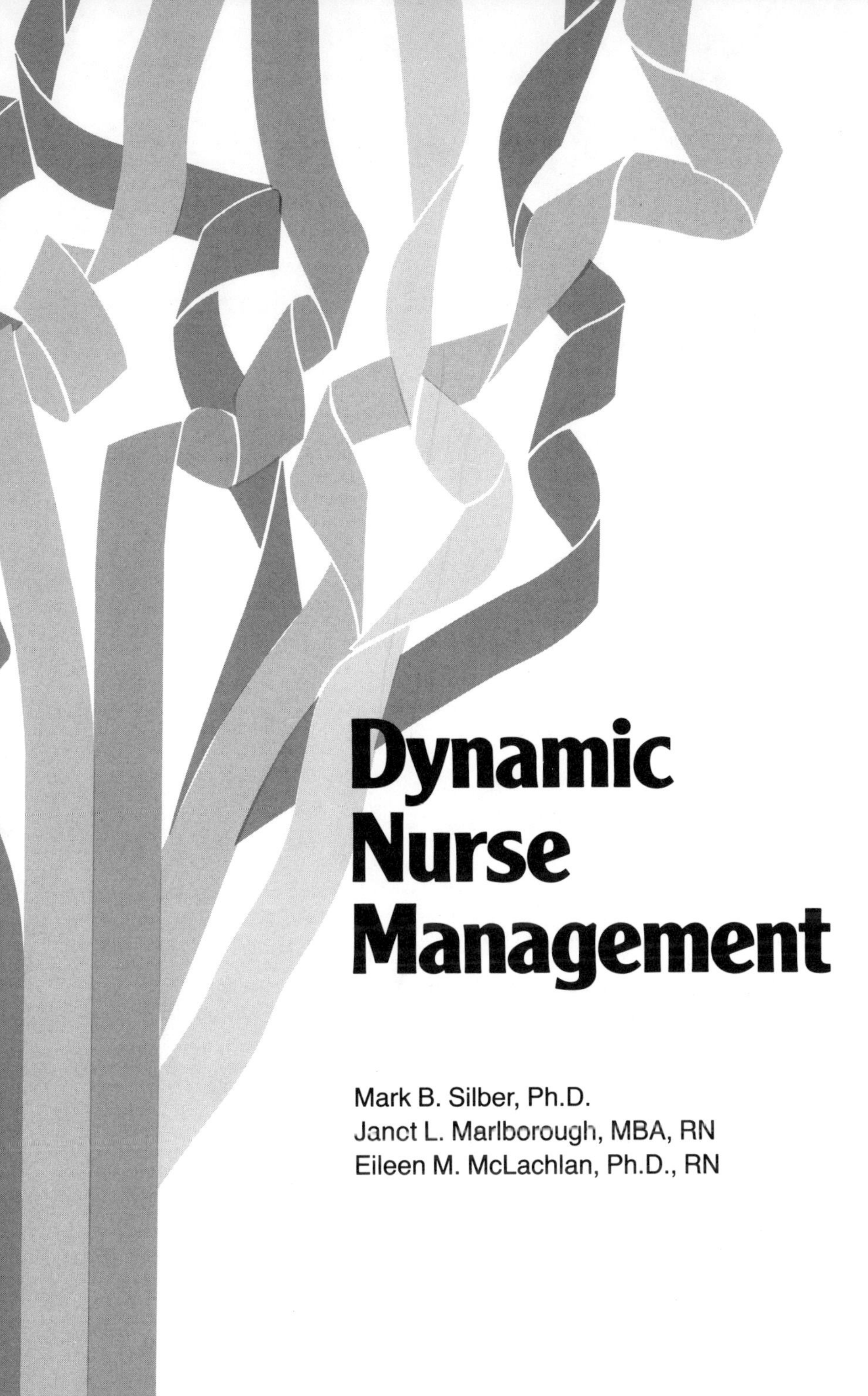

Dynamic Nurse Management

Mark B. Silber, Ph.D.
Janet L. Marlborough, MBA, RN
Eileen M. McLachlan, Ph.D., RN

Cabashon Publishing
Division of Health Education International, Inc.
11770 Bernardo Plaza Court, Suite 308
San Diego, California 92128

San Diego, Calif.: Cabashon Pub., © 1988P
Cabashon Pub.,
CURRENT PPD: 8802
Silber, Mark B.
Dynamic nurse management / Cabashon Pub., © 1988
ISBN: 0937825018 87-21862

Printed in the United States of America

To my wife Elizabeth, for being my companion in love as we travelled life's peaks and valleys and for her clinical insights as a nurse.

MBS

To all the nurses in today's health care system: the staff nurses, the managers, the strategic thinkers, the proactive persons, the teachers, the counselors, and all the others who are redefining the hospital from the bottom up.

JLM
EMM

Contents

Preface

Today's nursing management is complexity. From patient-care management to nursing administration, the complexities expanded geometrically in these last transitional years. Professional relationships between physicians and nurses have been redefined, and local, state, and federal governments have intervened with new legalities and restrictions. Today's economic and fiscal pressures are the realities of nurse management. The problems of economics *v* ethics—money *v* mission—compound the complexity. The gray areas of the biomedical ethics of professional practice are debated over a multitude of patient-care issues, but they remain clouded and unresolved.

Today's nursing management is complexity. The value systems of the work force are changing, staff members tend to have more education than ever before, and everyone seems to have more militant and sophisticated expectations. All these contribute to the complexity in manager-staff relations. Computerization, automation, and electronic technology of all kinds add to the confusion, and frustration may lead to a backlash of hostility and anger against "the system." In addition, the explosion of clinical and management knowledge has grown overwhelmingly in breadth and depth.

This complexity calls for an applied text that can assist all levels of nursing management in the quest to deal effectively with these dynamics and changing roles, relationships and responsibilities. This book presents a balanced selection of useful material that can provide increased insight into the contemporary nature of nurse-managers' "behaviors for results." What are the performance and productivity characteristics of nurse-managers who succeed in the real, real world of hospital politics, patient care and the new professional demands of clinical services? Why are some health care organizations running profitably, with vitality, while other hospitals, health maintenance organizations, and alternative-care facilities are faltering, and their brick and mortar are "the houses of the living dead"?

The performance objectives of this book are as follows:

1. To serve the reader by addressing the real and practical problems of managing with people on the units and eliciting cooperation between nursing and the other service support departments to get the tasks done

2. To produce a hands-on text that is a blend of management, research, and professional practice; covers substantive issues at both the individual and organizational level; and focuses on real-life dilemmas that nursing management must grapple with on the job

3. To show experienced clinical services directors, house supervisors, and newly appointed nurse managers how applied management psychology can aid them in their career climb and enhance their influence and impact on the organizational system

4. To design and develop a single text, albeit humbly and ambitiously, that addresses the relationships between experienced staff persons in today's hospitals—the interface between nurse-managers and empowered and motivated health care employees that can lead to job enrichment

5. To offer possible solutions from organizational psychology that managers might consider when facing the changing human and organizational complexities and costs in today's stressed health care profession

6. To better undergird the reader for management performance when the personal and political realities of professional life must be confronted

7. To promote the reader's personal examination of perceptions, human sensitivities and awareness as these affect professional and personal success within the microsociety or family called the health care system and to help the reader better deal with the human side of managing, the cognitive and emotional aspects of the persons with whom managers interact
8. To stimulate the reader's thoughtful consideration of the various topics and applied subjects chosen for the book
9. To combine thoroughness, enjoyable readability and thought-provoking information without falling into the trap of colorless writing and never-ending boring chapters of theory

This book was written and designed for use (1) in the core curricula of in-house management development and education and schools of nursing; (2) in seminars for multidiscipline health providers at both the university and community college levels and for schools of business administration; and (3) by those persons committed to progress in their upward career climb. It was written for individual study as well as for adaptation in courses of nursing management.

This joyful task of writing has taken 2 years. The various drafts of chapters have been written and edited in New Zealand, after shelling at Marco Island, while sitting on a rock overlooking the Maine coastline, on planes traveling to more than 200 hospital consulting assignments, in hotel rooms from Atlanta to Anaheim, and in the den of my home in sunny San Diego.

It is my fervent, fervent hope that this book will be not only up to date, but also pace-setting in guiding the development of both present and future nurse-managers as they go about their praiseworthy calling.

Mark B. Silber, PhD
San Diego, California
December 1987

Acknowledgments

We are grateful to you, the members of nursing management across the United States who not only have assisted us in seeing the necessity for this practical book but also, in your quest for continuous quality patient care, have provided the real purpose behind this book—the caring and curing of suffering human beings.

Our personal and professional appreciation is extended to the many directors of clinical services and the multitude of nurse managers at the client hospitals we have served as consultants. It is their on-the-firing-line insights that have added true value to our understanding of the realities of nursing management in these tough, turbulent and transitional times of health care.

MBS
JLM
EMM

It is with professional pride that I give full credit to my two remarkable and committed colleagues. Eileen McLachlan and Janet Marlborough are experienced nurse-managers and nurse-educators in their own right, and they were invaluable in the design and development of this book. Their competent insights into nurse management, faithful follow-through and indefatigable encouragement deserve affirmed and public gratefulness.

Authors often mistakenly think they are giants in the profession without the humble realization that they have gained their perceptions and vantage point by standing on the shoulders of those professional heavyweights who have assisted them in their growth. I acknowledge and am indebted to the many outstanding health care experts who have significantly influenced me—Kaiser, Peters, Deal, Herzberg, Maslow, Drucker, Fleishman, Lippitt, Feinberg, and a multitude of other health care professionals. Special acknowledgement is given to two persons who are "pro's pros" as behavioral scientists—Dr. Nancy Mansfield and Dr. V. Clayton Sherman. Thank you, Clay and Nancy, for your support and past co-authorships.

MBS
December 1987

Information on Continuing Education Credit

Ten hours of continuing education (CE) credit are available for this offering.

This self-paced educational program is sponsored by Health Education International, Inc. (HEI), which has been granted approval of its total program of continuing education credit in nursing by the Western Regional Accrediting Committee of the American Nurses' Association. HEI has been approved as a provider by the California Board of Registered Nursing (Provider No. 04960) and by the Florida Board of Nursing (Provider No. 2711004).

Continuing education credits may be obtained for reading this book. For further information, see the accompanying test booklet or contact:

Health Education International, Inc.
11770 Bernardo Plaza Court, Suite 308
San Diego, CA 92128
(619) 451-0342

Chapter 1

Today's Challenges: Goals in Transition

On July 20, 1986, Jube Shiver, Jr,[1] of the *Los Angeles Times* discussed problems confronting health care. Highlights of his article included the following:

After a decade of robust growth and record profits, the hospital industry has been hit with financial problems. Medicare, Medicaid and private insurance have restricted payments and clamped down on escalating medical fees. Hospital companies are also losing patients to health maintenance organizations and preferred-provider programs, which seek to provide lower-cost health-care services.

Capital-intensive service industries have been able to achieve significant cost savings by lobbying for government deregulation, computerizing many aspects of their operations and building more energy-efficient plants and equipment.

Hospitals also are beginning to experiment with new technology and better management after years of operating outside the arena of traditional supply-and-demand market forces. But progress has been slow.

For-profit hospitals have turned to more aggressive marketing as a way to generate new profits.

To lure expectant mothers to its maternity ward, a medical center offers champagne and lobster dinners to parents who choose the hospital for their delivery. The hospital also advertises on radio and in newspapers and holds

an annual health fair at which it offers free and low-cost
tests to community residents.

Recently this hospital knocked down the walls of its
little-utilized medical surgery unit in order to open a more
profitable physical rehabilitation unit.

These are but a few examples of the economic pressures
within the health care system that are challenging nursing. The
main consumers of health care—state and federal governments,
insurance companies, and health maintenance organizations
(HMOs)—are responsible for covering the costs of payment, providing information on what facilities to use, and determining to
what extent services will be given.

This indicates a change in direction. It is a new signpost that
tells nursing to balance patient-care cost with quality patient
care. This transition is causing an uneasiness, a crisis, that is
measured not by an uprising but by a lack of equilibrium.[2]

To explain this crisis, it is important to note that nursing is
part of an open system: It not only operates within its own confines but also depends on input from outside its own boundaries.[3]

The Health Care System

When viewed as part of the total health care system, nursing
becomes more than patient care. The hospital imports nurse
energy from the community, transforms it into patient-care
characteristics of the hospital, exports the recovering patient
back into the community, and then reenergizes the hospital
resources via the community's recognition of excellence in
patient care. That is, as every nursing unit takes in resources,
transforms them, and sends them into the larger system where
the psychologic, sociologic, and cultural aspects interact, uneven
degrees of tension and reciprocity exist despite the fact that everything in an open system is related to everything else.[4]

This crisis can be understood by thinking of it as a group of concentric rings (Fig. 1-1). The outermost circle applies pressure to the next circle inwards. In turn, the second circle applies more pressure to the next circle inwards and so on. The outermost circle is rising economic pressure. The next circle inward is the health care system. Inside that is the hospital administration and then the nursing administrator. Finally, the nurse-manager is in the innermost circle, feeling all the pressures from all the areas.

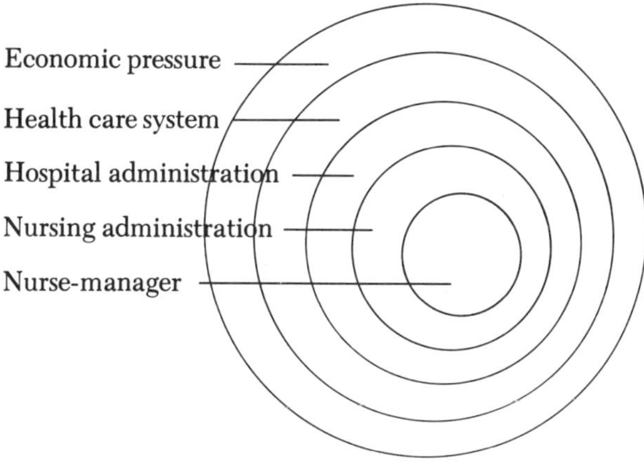

Figure 1-1—Schematic diagram of the crisis in the health care system.

The Old Signposts

All of these pressures demand that things be done differently, and as the pressures become more and more demanding, the familiar signposts of the health care system change. The signposts, the directions of traditional nursing, are familiar even to nursing students:

- Change the patients' sheets daily.

- Finish the patients' baths by 10 AM.
- Fill the patients' water pitchers by 9 PM.

These signposts were developed from the perspective of the patient as the consumer, and they remind us that for a long time nursing's immediate concern was the patient.

These signposts have been accepted as part of the nursing culture. Here are a few more that have pointed the way:

- All patients have the right to health care.
- Patients are always right.
- Patients have the right to ease and comfort.
- Patients can be hospitalized for as long as they wish.
- Care is personalized to suit the patients' needs.

These traditional signposts show how nursing has confined itself to a closed system in the name of patient-centered care. It has not kept alert to the changes in the hospital environment and the health care system. Although accrediting agencies have told nursing to look at its environment and build a team, nursing has continued to operate in isolation.

Denying interactions between other disciplines and itself, nursing has developed teamwork within the department to state-of-the-art proportions. Unfortunately, even staffing patterns for acuity have been developed without any ties to the finance and accounting departments. Thus, nursing has segregated itself as a culture in which mission, rather than management, has been favored heavily. Even the media portray nurses as altruistic, self-sacrificing caregivers who support the mission as the goal of priority.

Here is another example of mission as the preferred goal: When an emergency department (ED) nurse was confronted with lost dollars for supplies, her reply was, "I can't be bothered with accounting! We're here to save lives!" Technically, that nurse was correct. There is a time when the ED is very busy with tasks that take precedence over costing supplies. However, supply costs no longer can be ignored. That is to say, the goals of both mission and management always have been a part of nursing, but the management goal never has been a priority because a dollar value traditionally has not been attached to nursing care.

Because hospital administrations and nursing services have operated independently, the administration, without consulting nursing service, has raised the bed rates whenever it has been determined that a financial bind existed. A financial crisis has not been associated with or allocated to the cost of patient care. Traditionally, nurses never have been expected to be accountable for cost-effectiveness—their mission has been service. They have not been responsible for balancing the goals of patient-care services and patient-care costs.

Another traditional signpost is the reactive role of the nurse. A reactive nurse is affected by an event initiated by another, as in the case of a nurse waiting for the physician to initiate action for the patient. The nurse has been expected to respond to the patient and medical decisions and wait to be told the proper therapeutic techniques to use. This old signpost pointed in the right direction during an era when people came to the hospital to recover or to die. Now that there has been a shift to outpatient medicine and shorter hospital stays, these signposts are no longer familiar.

The New Signposts

New signposts have become familiar as technology has grown and medical and pharmaceutical techniques have developed. People come to the hospital for a new reason: the expert advice of the medical professional. Patients have grown accustomed to coming to the hospital for routine admissions, tests, and procedures as well as for surgical intervention.

However, economic forces have imposed new regulations on the health care system. To illustrate this, consider that in 1984 a major appliance division of a well-known company spent more on health care of their employees than on research and development of new products (personal communication). It does not take long to understand that major industry, such as this company, had to put a stop on rising health care costs and so devised appropriate actions by contracting for health care at a percentage of cost rather than total charges. Suddenly the hospital has had to take a critical look at the way it does business because the revenue stream has decreased. Lost revenue has had to be rebuilt by increasing patient volume and decreasing patient-care costs. This has changed the direction of nursing.

Other new signposts, new directions, will provide better financial security for the hospital. However, a problem does exist, and it is the antithesis to the traditional nurse-manager. Today's nurse-manager must be knowledgeable in business deals and must deal with optimal recovery guidelines, the greater severity of illness among patients, and an increase in patient volume—all in the context of higher productivity, greater efficiency, and high-quality care. The nurse-manager's directive is to lower costs of both labor and technology, but this can be misinterpreted.

For example, an editor of a major nursing journal decried the "rationing of nursing care" as nurses were forced to look at the costs of providing care.[5] She thought that the nurses actively rationed care to the patients, when, in reality, the only alternative to the nurse-manager was to decrease the costs for personnel. Nursing is a labor-intensive business. Because the highest costs are salaries, it behooves the nurse-manager to look ahead and find new solutions for increasing costs instead of throwing more money and more personnel at the problem.

In management terms, the nurse-manager must use both human and monetary resources to balance cost-effective goals with quality-care goals. The proactive nurse—one who initiates, directs, and is interdependent in actions—can make this possible.[6] A proactive nurse often may be described as an entrepreneur, one who takes on challenges, or one who takes on risk and makes things happen. An ED nurse can be proactive by deciding independently, after caring for a trauma patient, to determine the cost of the care by calculating service rendered and supplies used.

Proactive is a term that indicates anticipation of an event.[7] Sometimes experienced chief executive officers (CEOs) talk about using a "gut level" feeling to anticipate problems and make decisions. This intuitive behavior leads to strategic thinking that is a part of proactive management and defines a planning component.

Strategic thinking takes scanning behavior and develops a plan of action from it as it envisions a future different from the past. Strategic thinking is not foreign to nurses who continually scan their patients, watching for physiologic and psychologic changes. These nurses have developed the ability to satisfy needs. Now, they need to combine this craft with business skills to maintain and sustain a competitive advantage and to capitalize on the hospital's and nurses' strengths.

Strategic thinking is not reserved for the centralized level. It starts with the first-line supervisor, the head nurse. The head nurse sees the opportunities for achieving excellence when making rounds. This is the time to discuss with patients their reactions to hospitalization. Through individual interactions, positive as well as negative hospital experiences can be defined. Through discussions with the physicians to determine their reactions to patient care, the head nurse can determine improved ways for meeting physicians' expectations. Combining patients' needs and physicians' expectations into one plan of action can provide cost-effective, quality care that will meet the hospital's goal.

This does not mean that to be proactive a nurse must make decisions continually and initiate constantly. The term refers, instead, to a style of management.

Nurses who are successful with this style of management often are perceived as valuable assets. A physician recently asked why all the "good" nurses were leaving the floor for other departments. He described the "good nurses" as capable of making independent decisions and developing a level of trust. He was describing a proactive nurse.

Proactive nurse-managers are the ones who learn that they must have a finite grasp of financial effectiveness, the ability to clearly define financial responsibility, and the know-how to measure and implement an effective strategy for more productivity.

This defines another new demand of the nurse-manager who probably has been assigning staff members according to an acuity system that allows a team member a number of patients with a range of illness levels. Staffing for patients who are less ill balances the staffing for patients who are acutely ill. With the shortened length of hospital stay, many of the less sick patients are eliminated. This demands new staffing patterns, as the nurse-manager must arrange staffing for sicker patients who will stay for a shorter length of time. This makes nurse management an unusual business that is labor-intensive as well as technically intensive.

It takes management skills to guide nurses along the career path in nurse management, which starts with shift managers and continues with promotions to positions as floor managers, multiunit supervisors, and administrators. Although the positions are diverse, the path is narrow because nursing has not looked outside the profession for assistance in developing management style.

Nurses are educated to consider care of the patient a priority and graduate to the hospital setting where they are expected to combine it with cost-effectiveness. This introduces them to the two goals of hospital corporate culture: mission and management. When nurses discover the incongruence between their expectations about quality care as the priority and the demand for cost-effectiveness, reality shock sets in.[8]

Programs of nursing education have not begun to recognize the necessity of formal management skills in their curricula.[9] Ironically, an expectation of all new nurses, once they are hired by a hospital, is to "manage" either six patients or a nursing team.

Now, along with the demands of industry for changes in health care costs comes a demand for a change in patient care. The economic forces that have led health care costs on an escalating path now are changing the direction of nurse management. This change is causing a disturbance that can be recognized as crisis.

The Crisis

Crisis can be caused by the challenge that ensues from changes in responsibilities at work or from a change to a different line of work.[10] When a manager responds to such a challenge (speaking in business terms), the manager's level of anxiety rises, and four phases of a crisis emerge.[11] In the first phase the anxiety stimulates the manager's usual management skills. If these do not bring relief, and situational support is inadequate, the manager progresses to the second phase, which is even more anxious. In the third phase the manager tries out new management skills or redefines the challenge so that the old skills can work. Resolution can occur in this phase. If resolution does not occur, however, the manager goes on to the fourth phase in which the continuation of severe or panic levels of anxiety may lead to complete disorganization.

These phases of crisis should be considered in light of important balancing factors:[2] the manager's perception of the event, situational supports, and management skills. Successful resolution of the crisis is more likely if the manager's perception of the challenge is realistic rather than distorted, if situational supports are available so that others may help meet the challenge, and if the manager has the management skills to meet the challenge.

In other words, as the economic pressures impinge on the equilibrium of the health care system, a state of disequilibrium occurs. Along with this disequilibrium there is a perceived need to restore equilibrium. If one or more balancing factors are absent, the challenge will not be met. A distorted perception of today's financial challenge, lack of adequate situational support from peers and supervisors, and/or inadequate management skills will result in an unresolved problem—a situation that leads to further disequilibrium and crisis (Fig. 1-2).

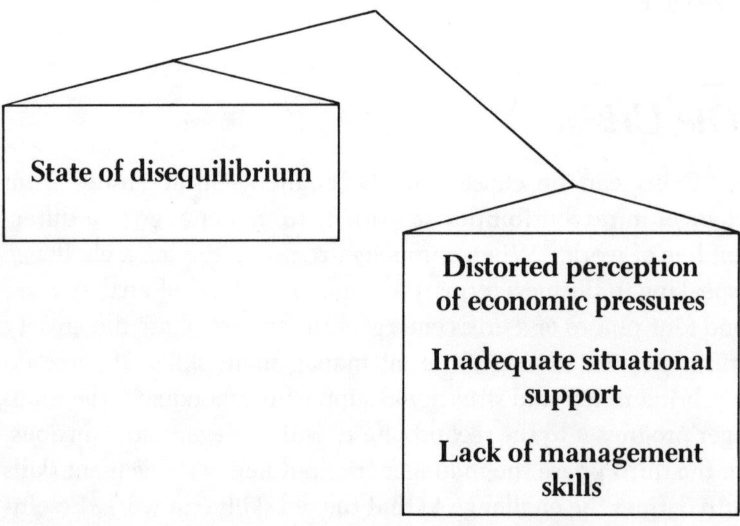

Figure 1-2—The Effects of Imbalancing Factors

Crisis Resolution

On the other hand, if one or more balancing factors are initiated, the present challenge will be met. With a realistic perception of the challenge, adequate situational support, and adequate management skills, the problem will be resolved, equilibrium will be regained, and there will be no crisis (Fig. 1-3).

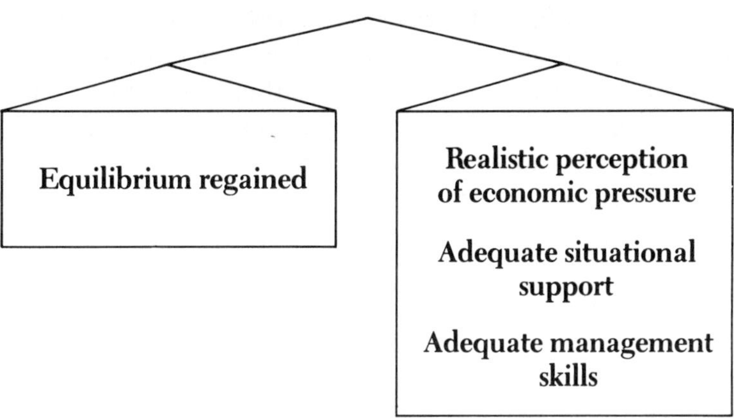

Figure 1-3—The Effects of Balancing Factors

In the past, nursing apparently viewed the goals of cost and care as mutually exclusive. The concern was that managing costs would succeed only at the expense of care. This generated much anxiety about how nurses could combine the mission of quality care for patients with the management of patient-care cost. This was a distorted perception of the challenge brought about by economic forces.

A more realistic perception of the challenge is that both mission and management are possible. As an example, the nurse can show cancer patients how to manage their own care by instructing them in care of the Hickman catheter, nutrition therapy, expected body changes, expected results of medication, signals of complications, and acceptance of the disease process. This makes it possible for the patient with cancer to have shorter stays in the hospital and longer stays at home. By teaching the patient what it takes for quality care at home, the nurse has taken the initiative to decrease hospitalization costs. The mission of nursing and the management of cost have been combined.

The second factor for resolving a crisis is developing a reliable system of support. When the nurse-manager works within a crisis situation while designing new staffing patterns and planning new budgeting and productivity systems, self-esteem may be threatened. Management effectiveness requires a feeling of adequacy as reinforced by a support group made up of peers or supervisors, but the nurse-manager often finds it too difficult to ask for help. Consequently, indirect communications emerge that give evidence of the nurse-manager's need for support. Often statements of ambivalence about staff members and dissatisfaction with their progress is a way of asking for help.

Because this call for help is hidden, the troubled nurse-manager frequently will get nods of agreement and no assistance from the peer group. On the other hand, when nurse-managers openly support one another and share styles, trials, and successes, then crisis can be resolved.

Resolving crisis situations also requires adaptive management skills. Shortened stays in the hospital for patients have made it necessary for the nurse to compress many tasks into a three-day span. The nurse-manager must think in terms of categories and outcomes of patient care while managing productivity systems, maintaining quality, assuming fiscal responsibility, and preserving flexible staffing. For a long time the value of a nurse, the caregiver, has been projected within the cost of the bed rate. Now, the nurse-manager must look at a return on investment (ROI) as a variable of human resource management even as staff members are hired.

Even though a nurse-manager may have had the opportunity to develop this kind of financial responsibility of determining a budget and planning capital acquisitions, evaluating the productivity of a unit and staff members in light of lost revenues or profit is difficult. This type of human resource management takes on new meaning when the nurse-manager is expected to translate the newly balanced goals for nursing, the mutually adaptive goals of mission and management, to staff members.

Staff members must have the new goals defined with an emphasis that the by-products of the new alliance between mission and management are quality care, decreased length of stay, and maximum productivity of the unit. When productivity is introduced, and every staff member is held accountable for maintaining a reduced staffing standard, staff members no doubt will grumble about it. And it will not be a surprise when patients hear that there is not enough help to answer a call bell quickly because the nurse-manager is working on productivity. Needless to say, staff members need an exact explanation of the plan for cost-effective, quality care.

They need to know that the census of hospitals in the United States is expected to drop about 15% each year. This will require development of cost-management protocols, use of home health agencies, and an understanding of intense care limited to very short hospital stays. To maintain patient days, to prevent a drop greater than the expected 15%, the volume of patients must be increased. Each staff member must recognize that to remain solvent, the hospital will have to increase the number of admissions while decreasing the length of time any one patient is hospitalized.

To be more specific, five fundamental managerial skills are needed to ensure success in meeting the challenges in today's health care world:

1. *Communication*, which helps analyze message units to formulate plans and operate strategies.
2. *Motivation*, which helps to gain the hospital's goals by matching them with the goals of staff members.
3. *Power-strategies*, which use influence to bring about change.
4. *Becoming a change agent*, which leads to the recognition that participation reduces resistance.
5. *Counseling*, which returns the problem employee to productivity.

In summary, the crisis in the health care system has developed through a series of relationships—a dynamic process.[6] It arises from disequilibrium between balancing factors. Crisis colors the interactions between departments, which are characterized in the behaviors of disorganization. However, this crisis may act as a positive force. Pressure from one side may force the other to evaluate perceptions of the challenge. Resolution of the crisis must be evaluated in terms of the overall success of the nursing organization.

Success often is measured by productivity, and productivity is measured in both qualitative and quantitative terms. For example, productivity will be achieved by matching staffing and supplies to volume, by matching nurses and supplies to lengths of hospitalization.

Success also is measured by stability, which is defined as keeping the turnover of human resources to a minimum. As turnover decreases, unit cohesiveness, motivation, and job identity increase.[12]

Additionally, success is measured by adaptability to internal and environmental pressures. The nurse-manager who can adapt to these pressures is singled out as a team player. In other words, crisis forces an evaluation in terms of successes and failures. If nurse-managers are to be successful, they must improve productivity, strive for stability, adapt to the changing environment, and resolve crisis.

Because of the challenge by economic forces, every nurse-manager must know the impact of the changing hospital on the staff; recognize that effort towards achievement, not activity, guarantees effectiveness; and develop adequate management techniques. These three concepts—the changing hospital, the effective manager, and fundamental managerial skills—are the basis for this book.

Chapter 2, "The Changing Hospital," discusses the new information-rich, decentralized, technologic hospital in which creativity gives an edge to competition. It describes how performance can be influenced by climate and how culture makes for an outstanding continuous performance.

Chapter 3, "The Effective Manager," contains specific tactics to be used and ways to counteract negative reactions. It lists specific ways to improve practice to a peak performance and discusses negotiation, leadership, and conflict resolution.

The process of communication, organizational communication, and the application of communication strategies form the content of chapter 4.

Chapter 5 stresses how the nurse-manager's need to recognize the improving performance in hospitals is related directly to how well persons are motivated through meaningful work.

Chapter 6 describes five sources of power and a method for developing personal power strategies to become a power-projecting person.

A specific plan for change and ways to overcome resistance are the core of chapter 7.

Chapter 8 describes three specific types of counseling for the problem employee and how retraining or transferring may be the way to reconcile the employee within the working unit.

After a broad overview of social and economic history, chapter 9 describes an awareness of the new value system, a development of the art of followership, the definition of motivators, the identification of dissatisfiers, the initiation of open communication, and the recognition of empowerment skills.

Most of this book focuses on helping nurses learn ways to develop management skills. The basic belief is that nurses can become more effective managers by increasing their understanding of culture, communication, motivation, power, change, and counseling. These concepts can help nurses face today's challenges and tomorrow's changes.

References

1. Shiver J Jr: Health firms go under the budget knife. *Los Angeles Times*, July 20, 1986, part IV, p 1.
2. Aguilera DC, Messick JM: *Crisis Intervention: Theory and Methodology*, ed 3. St Louis, The CV Mosby Co, 1978.
3. Katz DL, Kahn RL: Organizations and the system concept, in *The Social Psychology of Organizations*, ed 2. New York, John Wiley & Sons Inc, 1978, pp 17-34.
4. Perrow C: The short and glorious history of organizational theory. *Organizational Dynamics*. AMACOM, Summer 1973. As found in Gibson JL, Ivancevich JM, Donnelly JH, (eds): *Readings in Organizations*. Plano, Tex, Business Publications Inc, 1982, pp 32-43.
5. Kelly L: When nurses ration care. *Nurs Outlook* 1985;33:123-124.
6. Marguiles N, Raia AP: *Organizational Development: Values, Process, and Technology*. New York, McGraw-Hill Book Co, 1972.
7. Odiorne G: *The Change Resisters*. Englewood Cliffs, NJ, Prentice-Hall Inc, 1981.
8. Kramer M: *Reality Shock*. St Louis, The CV Mosby Co, 1974.
9. McLachlan E: *Perceived Role Expectations for Associate and Baccalaureate Degree Nurses*, doctoral dissertation. United States International University, San Diego, Calif, 1984.
10. Stuart GW, Sundeen SJ: *Principles and Practices of Psychiatric Nursing*. St Louis, The CV Mosby Co, 1979.
11. Caplan G: *Principles of Preventive Psychiatry*. New York, Basic Books Inc Publishers, 1964.
12. Hickman CR, Silva MA: *Creating Excellence*. New York, The New American Library Inc, 1984.

Chapter 2

The Changing Hospital

Like a human being, hospitals go through change as they adjust both internally and externally to the various environments that nurture their survival. Through these changes, hospitals, like humans, may become rigid and deteriorate in their ability to deliver service. Those that remain ongoing, that focus on regularly changing the environment, continue to achieve and mature. Often though, struggling hospitals are so busy facing crisis in the external environment that they neglect to make internal changes. Yet, these are the very changes necessary to meet a competitive environment, to cope with conflict, and to respond to new requirements in health services.

The Changing Environment

Recent developments in the competitive health care marketplace, the changed corporate culture of the hospital and its impact on the staff, are the preoccupations of reality. Nurse-managers know that the nursing profession is being challenged. Changes are forcing choices and tough decisions in these turbulent times.

Time-tested ways of making sense of the hospital world seem increasingly irrelevant. The old ways of thinking are being replaced by the new ways of understanding.[1] The high cost of care has reduced the hospital stay to a minimum. It no longer is possible for a patient to stay indefinitely in the hospital to receive maximum treatment for the healing process. Shortened hospital stays have changed the patient's role from that of a dependent person to that of a partner in health. Hospitals have become decentralized systems with satellite care centers to serve the community better. To cut down on hospitalizations, the goal of care has changed from one of eliminating disease to one of promoting well-being. Table 2-1 succinctly summarizes these changes.

Idea	Old Way	New Way
Goal	Eliminate disease	Promote well-being
Body	Machine needing repair	Dynamic system
Patient	Dependent	Partner
Therapy	Maximum	Minimum
Pain	Negative	Information
Responsibility	Physician	Self (patient)
Health system	Centralized	Decentralized

Table 2-1—The Changing Environment in Health Care

Source: Adapted with permission from Pointer DD: Preparation for the new age. Hosp Forum, November/December 1984, p 60.

These changes have significant implications as the focus of nursing increasingly becomes health—not illness. Accordingly, nurses will have to rethink their profession, to see it as one of keeping patients healthy and getting paid to do so. Pointer's insight[1] suggests that the successful medical center of the future will be one in which the consumer and the health organization share incentives and risks for staying well. This requires that the care process be redefined to include increasing amounts of self-care.

Ferguson[2] recognized this drive for self-care as a part of a social transformation that she called the "Aquarian conspiracy."

This new way of thinking about health conveys a message of hope and charges the individual with personal responsibility. The home and family have become the means to a secure but less costly recovery period. The family link has become so vital in the recovery process that recently surgeons denied a heart transplant to a baby whose parents were not married. Not until temporary custody was given to the paternal grandparents and family stability guaranteed could the heart transplant be considered. This new way of health delivery enlarges the framework of the old as it incorporates brilliant technologic advances.

As technology took a central role in modern medical care, computerized blood analyzers, tomography scanners, renal dialysis machines, cardiac monitors, and even organ transplants became expected available services for any person admitted to a hospital. The development and wide-spread use of expensive medical technologies is one of the main reasons for the sharp increase in health costs.

At one time it made good sense to keep the labor force healthy regardless of cost, so corporations offered health insurance as an employee benefit. As long as health costs were met by the insurance plan or government agencies on a cost-plus basis, there was no need to be concerned.

However, as health costs skyrocketed, providing health care became one of the highest costs of doing business. The annual corporate health bill has now reached $100 billion.[3] That is $100,000,000,000! In 1983 the United States spent 11 % of its gross national product (GNP) on health care, whereas in 1960 it spent only 5.3 %. Thus, the annual cost of health care soared from $27 billion in 1960 to $360 billion in 1983, and by the year 2000 money spent on health care is expected to be 15 % of GNP.

Until recently, when persons needed medical treatment, they got it. There were no questions asked. However, for a government faced with an absolutely appalling deficit or for companies faced with the costs of health insurance as one of the most expensive items in their operations budgets, the cost of health care had to be decreased.

In 1983 it was the federal government that blew the whistle by announcing that the amount of money Medicare would pay for various procedures would be limited and paid on the basis of diagnosis-related groups (DRGs). With DRGs the hospital had to control costs.

Now, corporations are trying out new ways to control health costs. As described by Naisbitt and Aburdene,[4] these new ways include the following:

1. All health costs are being audited.
2. Medical experts are being hired to monitor treatment of employees.
3. Business groups are determining the most cost-effective hospitals.
4. Corporations are building their own on-site medical facilities.
5. Companies are paying health claims themselves.
6. HMOs are being used because they offer fees that range from 10% to 40% less than an insurance premium.
7. Corporations are joining preferred-provider organizations (PPOs) to link companies that want lower health care costs with hospitals that want more patients.
8. Minor emergencies are being sent to freestanding emergency centers.
9. Patients who need minor surgery are being encouraged to use ambulatory surgicenters because home recovery is cost-effective.
10. Companies are demanding smoke-free environments.
11. Wellness, health, and well-being are being promoted by the companies.

As might be expected, these changes require that all members of the nursing profession and all hospital personnel, from inside and outside, from top to bottom, think differently. Hospitals need to heed Curtin's advice[5]:

1. Actively encourage innovation by removing departmental obstacles such as bureaucracy, endless reviews, and chain of command.
2. Provide internal programs, funding, and time for new projects and ideas.
3. Let each department set its own goals to increase cost-effective productivity.
4. Pay attention to suggestions from the staff.
5. Get rid of the deadwood and demand progress.
6. Publicly recognize innovative individual achievements.
7. Cushion innovators from risks even when projects might not succeed.

Accomplishing these goals along with creative thinking and ingenious strategies can lead to the redesign of the complex hospital system, the appropriate reward of workers, a fair return on investment—and, ultimately, the reinvention of the hospital.

Signs of Changes

Signs of changes are already visible. Hospitals have fewer employees since Medicare and Medicaid were established in the late 1960s. When these programs permitted separate charges for bits and pieces of nurses' jobs, many technicians were employed. Now that separate charges no longer can be made or justified, the trend is towards hospitals having only registered nurses on staff. To eliminate layers of management, small units have been consolidated into large ones, and supervisors are responsible for one type of service regardless of location (eg, the maternal-child supervisor oversees the nursery, labor, and delivery, postpartum care, pediatrics, and the pediatric intensive care unit). To decrease the number of staff personnel, positions have been eliminated. The number of employees now depends on a standard based on the average-adjusted number of occupied beds.

Productivity measures have been instituted to hold staff

members accountable for output. For instance, in a home health agency the nurses were expected to make five home visits each day. To increase the capacity of staff personnel, each member is now cross-trained. If a cardiac technician is not available to draw blood for blood gases, the registered nurse can do it.

Budgets have been examined carefully, and any items not directly connected to patient care have been eliminated. Days off for continuing education courses have been eliminated. The pharmacy formulary has been reduced, which means that the stock on hand and the choices for prescription drugs are limited. Job expectations have been increased by instituting employee merit reviews that are based on performance rather than seniority.

Guidelines for Continuing Changes

Now that hospitals are engaged in a time of transformation, they must consider ways that can help them continue to grow and maintain their status within the community. Naisbitt and Aburdene[4] listed 10 considerations in reinventing the corporation. These can be paraphrased into terms for reinventing hospital management:

1. Hospitals that create the most nourishing environments for personal growth are attracting the most talented people.
2. Inside the hospital, the nurse-manager's new role is to cultivate and maintain the nourishing environment for personal growth.
3. Compensation systems that reward performance and innovation are transforming employees.
4. There is a shift from hired labor to contract labor, which is part of a larger trend to go outside the organization for a variety of support services.
5. The top-down authoritarian management style is

yielding to a matrix style of management. In this matrix employees learn from one another horizontally, everyone is a resource person, and each person gets support and assistance from many directions.

6. Many hospitals are changing the configuration of their corporate structure and creating subsidiaries that operate under the main tent of the corporation.
7. In the reinvented hospital, quality is expected.
8. ROI is gaining a new respectability in the hospital.
9. Hospitals are discovering that they must compete in a market-driven rather than a product-driven system.
10. Today's hospitals or satellites are being located where the most creative people can offer quality care to a new market.

Hospital Operations

Hospitals represent a special case of management performance because they must operate as for-profit entities and gain net revenues from patient care facilities for patients as well as from affiliated businesses. Management performance depends on establishing a clear mission that includes long-term business goals.

Nowadays hospitals have many alternative choices for their mission. Some choose to provide a place where physicians work. Others choose to be community centers that exist to protect the people in the immediate geographic area. Still others choose to define themselves as centers of excellence, such as burn centers, trauma units, or cardiac recovery units. Although the community is served best when different hospitals have different missions, quality of care is likely to be greatest in institutions that plan a special service and have large enough numbers of patients in that subspecialty to cover costs and provide a profit.[6]

Problems in Hospital Planning

According to Drucker,[7] planning is the continuous process of making risk-taking decisions systematically and with the best possible knowledge of their futurity, organizing systematically the efforts needed to carry out those decisions, and measuring the results of those decisions against the expectations through organized, systematic feedback. Unfortunately, the hospital has many problems in planning.

It is difficult to forecast economic change as it is related to market share because even though the numbers of patients served remain the same, reimbursement often is decreased. This means that the numbers of patients served must be increased, and length of stay must be decreased for the hospital to be profitable.

Another management problem is collection delay. Hospitals collect payments due to them slowly and have many write-offs. Any delay in collecting payment can upset a hospital's net operating income. To increase collections, counselors explain the cost of treatment beforehand and assist patients in planning a schedule for reimbursement.

Each department in a hospital is really a cost center, which means that the least amount of services provided results in the best ratio of cost to charges. Some departments do not generate enough revenues to carry the costs of the department. The answer to higher productivity is to offer the services that generate the most volume in the profitable units and drop the units that are used infrequently or serve the lowest number of patients.

Hospitals operate under the heavy costs of direct labor, expensive equipment, and highly paid specialists. In the past, hospitals ran some of their departments at a loss. Customary charges for those departments were lower than actual cost. When reimbursement is either at a break-even point or at a loss, cost structures should be revised to make customary charges higher than cost so that the department will break even.

The emphasis is that cost-effective planning can enhance hospital performance by doing the following:

- Increasing the number of patients served while decreasing the length of time they stay in a hospital
- Increasing collections
- Planning in advance for reimbursements
- Eliminating any departments that are used infrequently
- Revising cost structure so that charges are higher than cost

---

Performance and Organizational Climate

Hospital performance also is influenced by climate: the perceptions employees have about their organization's practices and operating principles. More specifically, climate is the way managers and other employees perceive the mixture of formal and informal policies, structures, and systems that guide management behavior and influence overall organizational performance. These perceptions are the result of interactions between an organization's structure and the character of its personnel. Climate is an expression of the prevailing value system.

A positive climate encourages participation in management. Welsch and Lavan[8] studied upper- and middle-management employees in a health care company and found that a participative climate was related to organizational commitment. Sense of teamwork was related to satisfaction with work and promotional opportunities.

The most satisfactory climate for productivity and job satisfaction is one that stresses achievement, positive motivation, involvement in goal setting, and a sense of individual responsibility. Nash,[6] listed eight climate factors:

1. Organizational clarity
2. Decision-making structure
3. Organizational integration
4. Management style
5. Performance orientation
6. Organizational vitality
7. Compensation
8. Development of human resources

Organizational clarity is a sharply outlined, distinct understanding of the organization's goals. It is present when people perceive the company's mission, objectives, processes, and activities as purposeful, rational, and fully communicated. This understanding acts as a unifying influence and enhances cooperation.

The term decision-making structure describes the process of rationally choosing a course of action from a group of alternatives and then implementing and systematically evaluating that choice. Decisions are perceived as relevant, rational, and effective.

Organizational integration is the extent to which various units cooperate and communicate to achieve the overall objectives of the organization. When organizational integration exists, employees believe that departments understand one another's objectives, needs, and problems and that communication, cooperation, and collaboration exist.

Management style is the pattern of delegated authority and employees' perceptions of freedom and constraint. A positive climate encourages managers to be free to determine and take actions they believe necessary to perform their jobs well.

Performance orientation is the degree of emphasis placed on accountability for clearly defined results and high levels of performance. In a positive climate employees know their accountabilities and standards of performance.

Organizational vitality is the extent to which employees perceive the organization's activity. A positive climate relays the message that the organization is dynamic, responsive to change, venturesome, and innovative.

Compensation is the perception about rewards and their availability. The climate is positive when the employees perceive compensation as equitable, competitive, and related to performance.

Development of human resources is the opportunity to develop a person's potential. When employees perceive that they have opportunities within the company to develop their potential, they reflect an organization that has high morale.

When these climate factors are positive, in any organization, long-term profitability, growth, and high morale will be the result. These behavior patterns are the expressed values of an organization's culture.

Organizational Culture

Every organization has a culture. It may be fragmented and difficult to read from the outside. It may be strong and cohesive. Whether it is weak or strong, culture has a powerful impact on any organization.

Culture, according to Webster's dictionary,[9] is the "integrated pattern of human behavior that includes thought, speech, action, and artifacts and depends on man's capacity for learning and transmitting knowledge to succeeding generations." Bower[10] offered a more succinct definition: "It's the way we do things around here."

According to Deal and Kennedy,[11] organizations that have cultivated strong individual identities by shaping values help their employees do their jobs a little better in two ways:

1. A strong culture is a system of informal rules that spells out how persons are to behave most of the time. When employees know exactly what is expected of them, little time is wasted in deciding how to act.

2. A strong culture enables employees to feel better about what they do, so they are more likely to work harder. When structure, standards, and a value system are provided, uncertainty about job expectations is removed.

Because every organization needs a strong culture, the ultimate success of management depends to a large degree on an accurate reading of the culture and the ability to hone it and shape it to fit the shifting needs of the marketplace. To paraphrase, the ultimate success of a nurse-manager depends to a large degree on an accurate reading of the hospital culture and the ability to sharpen the staff into a shape that fits the shifting needs of the health care system. Peters and Waterman[12] found that the most successful "excellent" managers were those who strived to make a mark by creating a guiding vision, shaping shared values, and otherwise providing leadership for persons with whom they worked.

Now is the time for tough-minded rethinking about hospital culture, for reaffirmation of nursing values, and for rededication of the nursing mission. Changes should be faced as opportunities, not obstacles. Cost-producing nursing practices should be removed. Cost-productive nursing should be encouraged. The key emphasis is on adjusting to the new health care system and helping the staff members understand the change.

Making these changes starts with the nurse-manager who is influential in creating a climate of understanding. Most nurse-managers will survive these changes; others will not be able to make the difficult transition. Nurse-managers can become performance leaders and be politically visible. Changing the system and creating a climate are management's choices and they are shaped by culture.

Culture and the Nurse-Manager

A hospital culture is a belief system that extends throughout nursing. This interpersonal fabric is not passive. It is a living, working element that permeates the health care system. Nurse-managers have the opportunity, as never before, to influence the development and powerful perpetration of a viable and vital culture.

The core of culture is the belief system that emphasizes the human dimension of nursing. The guiding themes in a vital nursing culture are the ideas that nurses are important persons and that nurses are winners. Treating persons effectively is the key to an integrated pattern of an enlightened culture. Nurse-managers can enhance and enrich the hospital culture by creating an environment that nurtures and cultivates the growth of staff members. The staff members then transmit these values of nurturance and growth to patients and colleagues. What evolves is a sharing milieu in which everyone is caught up in projecting core values.

Seven behavior patterns can transmit these core values:

C	Creating a climate
U	Understanding oneself
L	Leading
T	Trusting
U	Using communication
R	Recognizing rites and rituals
E	Expecting excellence

Creating a Climate

The *C* in culture reminds a nurse-manager of the opportunity to create a climate. Just as an agar plate culture within a laboratory setting requires a certain nurturing climate to attain growth, so does the progressive development of a hospital culture. When a hospital is viewed as a medium in which growth is expected from every employee, the challenge towards optimal achievement is impressive. The nurse-manager has a direct impact on releasing a tremendous reservoir of professional and hospital identification for the benefit of the hospital and for the reward that comes from individual maturing and growing within the self.

To stimulate this growth climate, the nurse-manager can determine underlying themes and capitalize on "organization scripts" that will guide staff members towards positive group feeling. An example of a bonding or linking theme comes from the often used hospital word "care." When the concept of care emanates from the nurse-managers as an operationalized value, then staff members will feel cared for. As care permeates the staff in the hospital environment, care will be projected to the patients in the hospital environment. In this way care has the pervasive potential of being reinforced repeatedly.

Each nurse-manager transmits the care value by encouraging supportive relations in all units. What counts is that the nurse-manager is a visible, influencing force in perpetuating this value. From examples of a supportive presence, this action-demonstrated value can be extended by a manager who creates a climate of caring.

Understanding Oneself

The *U* in culture is understanding oneself. The need for nurse-managers to understand themselves is important in the culture-cultivating process. The ability to influence depends on healthy self-esteem. Nurse-managers who have positive self-esteem take periodic inventory of their abilities and shortcomings. They know who they are and who they are not. They realize that they have within themselves the power to make enhancing decisions. Nurse-managers with high self-esteem use their influential power to manage themselves first.

To provide a framework of management competencies, Boyatzis[13] grouped management skills into these categories: actions, human resources, leadership, focus on others, supervising, and knowledge.

Action skills indicate an ability to make things happen:

- Thinking in terms of both improving and removing things to do
- Supporting requests that facilitate staff members' productivity
- Putting problems or crises into solvable frameworks
- Listening to upper management, peers, and staff

Human resource skills emphasize work done through people:

- Supporting the team player regardless of a personal need for power
- Believing that persons are unique as individuals and have positive attributes
- Trusting persons to solve their own problems
- Founding and forming an influence base through others

Leadership skills indicate positive self-esteem:

- Communicating in an effective and acceptable manner
- Realizing that thinking and actions must be consistent and focused
- Recognizing that problems are defined from many facts

Skills of focusing on others include a psychologic sensitivity and the ability to relate socially to others:

- Controlling personal needs, emotions, and fears
- Seeing the other side of discussions and debates
- Demonstrating positive reciprocity by being comfortable with others and having others be comfortable with management

Supervising skills indicate an ability to guide others:

- Reaching out to others
- Getting things done by using a power base
- Expressing thoughts and emotions with comfort

Knowledge skills show the ability to accumulate specialized information:

- Keeping up to date on nursing practices and philosophy

Understanding nurse-managers, then, depend on action, use of human resources, leadership, an ability to focus on others, guidance, and up-to-date knowledge.

Leading

The *L* in culture stands for leading people with effectiveness. According to Drucker,[7] effectiveness is doing the right things that make a real difference in an organization. Nurse-managers lead by listening to staff members and treating them with respect. They provide an open-door policy of political safety, interact with staff members, and share frequent and honest feedback.

Trusting

The *T* in culture stands for trusting, with an emphasis on *us*. Nurse-managers trust employees to produce success. The common value of trust binds staff and management together in their individualized and joint efforts.

In a trusting atmosphere, nurse-managers convey by actions and attitude that their job is not to control persons, but to control progress. They give staff members political visibility, facilitating attendance at meetings that can give other staff members authority and freedom to make decisions. Nurse-managers listen to suggestions from staff members and observe personal abilities and values. They trust the problem-solving ability of staff personnel.

Using Communication

The second *U* in culture reminds nurse-managers to use the communication network. Communication up and down the hospital hierarchy does not depend on memoranda and notes to spread orders. Each hospital has an informal network that presumes that every employee takes an unofficial role in communicating changing events. Deal and Kennedy[11] recognized the following functions of communication:

1. Clarifying organizational history
2. Defining beliefs in terms of past precedents
3. Providing a boost for young personnel when they are frustrated by change

Thus, nurse-managers who have been present during the growth years of the hospital can clarify the hospital history by being an observer of changes, define beliefs for care in terms of past precedents, and provide a boost for young graduate nurses when they are shocked by the reality of the changing hospital goals. Nurse-managers use the grapevine.

Recognizing Rites and Rituals

The *R* in culture stands for recognizing rites and rituals. The rites and rituals of a hospital show how and why things are done. Behind all the practices lies the informal legacy of a hospital culture that represents the sources of value and meaning. Each ritual provides a framework for action. Whether it is nurses listening to the "morning report" or physicians eating in the "private dining room," these rituals reveal the expectations of the traditional hospital. Computer printouts and taped messages from the previous shift show a new trend in morning reports that might develop into a ritual of a changing hospital. These rites and rituals can define the type of hospital culture and signal a bureaucratic or collegial climate. Nurse-managers recognize what the rites and rituals indicate and sense the influence that can be expected when these rites and rituals are incorporated into group action.

Expecting Excellence

The final letter in culture, *E*, stands for expecting excellence. When nurse-managers expect excellence, they provide staff members with a climate for excellent service and self-satisfying achievement. Excellence can be achieved by means of a consistent belief on the part of each nurse-manager that persons want to become what they are capable of becoming.

In their book, *In Search of Excellence*, Peters and Waterman[12] focused on these core values for achieving excellence:

1. Worth and value of people
2. Service, care, and concern
3. Follow-through quality
4. Informality

All of these values revolve around people. Nurse-managers recognize that people are the ones who achieve quality and productivity. People are the means to cost-effective innovation. People bring about change by "non-scared" thinking, probing analysis, and commitment to action. Nurse-managers encourage and expect excellence.

New Skills for the Nurse

What do nurse-managers need to know about new skills for the staff nurse? To paraphrase Naisbitt and Aburdene,[4] the hospital's competitive edge is nurses—an educated, skilled work force who are eager to develop their human potential while contributing to the growth of the health care system. Yet, evidence is growing that nurse graduates joining the hospital's work force are less skilled than ever before—less skilled in technologic know-how and uninformed about the "high-tech/high-touch" formula. Nurses need to know that whenever technology is introduced, it must be counterbalanced with the human response of high-touch.

Nurses have known for a long time that their educational system did not prepare them for the reality of hospital expectations. Naisbitt and Aburdene[4] have declared that it is time to give nurses some TLC, which does not mean tender loving care. It stands for thinking, learning, and creating. Technology has brought with it a dearth of easily accessible information. "The dilemma is that there is never enough time to teach all the information that could usefully be taught."[4] The more information nurses have, the more they need to be competent thinkers.

Thinking is the ability to synthesize and make generalizations, to divide into categories, to draw inferences, to distinguish between fact and opinion, to put facts in order to analyze a problem. According to de Bono,[14] "Thinking has to do with the way information is arranged and rearranged to make decisions, solve problems, create opportunities and raise human potential. Thinking is the most fundamental and important skill and it *can* be learned and developed."

In the hospital that is constantly changing, no one subject or set of subjects will serve the nurses for the foreseeable future, let alone for the rest of their lives. The most important skill is learning how to learn. If nurses know how to learn, they can adapt and change no matter what changes come in pediatric, obstetric, medical, or surgical nursing skills. Nurses no longer can rely on segregated specialized skills. Nursing requires learning an integrated approach.

How then will nurses learn? Because learning requires openness and curiosity, they will have to learn first "how to unlearn." (Facts and answers cannot always be given.) Because learning requires humility, they will have to be able to concede that there are others better and more clever than they. (Technicians with specialized education may have the answer.) Because learning requires exploring, they will learn many things by trial and error. (They will be given the privilege to be wrong.)

In a place where routines, uniformity, and centralization have existed for so long, creativity has not been a value. In this new information-rich, decentralized, technologic hospital, however, creativity can give an edge to competition. The new marketing environment of the hospital requires this special talent. Gone are the days when mass production relied on uniformity to aid production. Now is the time for management to discover effectiveness through creativity.

As labor-effective organizations, hospitals need to use thinking, learning, and creativity to hone their staff into a competitive edge for quality care. It is sharp competition that carves a spot in the health care marketplace. How the staff nurses are guided and motivated toward the hospital's new mission—high quality, cost-effective care—depends on effective managers.

References

1. Pointer DD: Preparation for the new age. *Hosp Forum*, November/December 1984, pp 60-61.
2. Ferguson M: *The Aquarian Conspiracy*. Los Angeles, JP Tarcher Inc, 1980.
3. Naisbitt J: *Megatrends*. New York, Warner Books Inc, 1982.
4. Naisbitt J, Aburdene P: *Re-inventing the Corporation*. New York, Warner Books Inc, 1985, pp 181-202.
5. Curtin LL: Re-inventing the hospital. *Nurse Management*, November 1985, pp 10-11.
6. Nash M: *Managing Organizational Performance*. San Francisco, Jossey-Bass Inc Publishers, 1983 pp 71-75.
7. Drucker P: *The Practice of Management*. New York, Harper & Row Publishers Inc, 1954.
8. Welsch HP, Lavan H: Inter-relationships between organizational commitment and job characteristics, job satisfaction, professional behavior, and organizational climate. *Human Relations* 1981;34:1079-1089.
9. *Webster's New Collegiate Dictionary*. Springfield, Mass, G & C Merriam Co, 1973, p 274.
10. Bower M: *The Will to Manage*. New York, McGraw-Hill Book Co, 1966.
11. Deal TE, Kennedy AA: *Corporate Cultures*. Menlo Park, Calif, Addison-Wesley Publishing Co Inc, 1982.
12. Peters TJ, Waterman RJ Jr: *In Search of Excellence*. New York, Warner Books Inc, 1982.
13. Boyatzis RE: *The Competent Manager*. New York, John Wiley & Sons Inc, 1982.
14. de Bono E: *Learning to Think*. New York, Capra Press, 1982.

Chapter 3

The Effective Nurse-Manager

The effective nurse-manager focuses time and attention on opportunities rather than on problems. Effectiveness resides in the ability to direct resources by pinpointing the efforts of staff members toward opportunities for the delivery of quality care. Furthermore, according to Drucker,[1] the effective manager focuses on doing the right things, whereas the efficient manager focuses on doing things right. The difference is that doing right things focuses on achievement, whereas doing things right focuses on movement and motion. Putting the effort towards achievement, not activity, enables the effective nurse-manager to make something happen for the goals of the organization.

Process Thinking

The goal-oriented nurse-manager is concerned with process (doing good rather than looking good). To develop process thinking requires open communication with staff members, a technique that involves risk taking on the part of the manager. It is easier for a nurse-manager to function without risk in a status quo environment. However, in a status quo environment, staff members decrease their initiative, their own personal risk taking, and their feedback, events that let the manager assume all the directives as well as all the risks. When staff members wait for signs from the nurse-manager before taking action, they leave all the decisions and risk taking to the manager.

The management of risk taking, or entrepreneurial innovation is the very heart and core of management.[1] It is in this light
that the effective nurse-manager spends a large percentage of
time away from the telephone in open communication with the
staff, identifying daring ideas and possible opportunities for progressive advancement for the hospital.

The effective nurse-manager invests time rather than spending it. The monetary value of time must be determined on the
basis of overhead, space, benefits, and salaries for the manager
and staff. Time, along with money and people, is part of the
scarce resources that must be managed within a hospital. When
nurses mismanage time, they mismanage their effectiveness.

Nurse-managers need to eliminate noncontributing procedures that dissipate time and waste resources. Nothing will
decrease effectiveness more than procedures that take too much
time. However, to eliminate routine behaviors is not a popular
move by managers. Therefore, the staff members and the manager need to come to a satisfactory agreement before changing
any routines.

Because management is defined as the ability to get results
through other people, the nurse-manager must allow staff members the freedom to get results by providing them the opportunity to solve their own problems. The nurse-manager removes
obstacles and develops strategies and tactics to decide on the best
solution. The manager provides the direction and clears the way.

An effective nurse-manager is a sounding board for solutions
that staff members may suggest for problems. The manager does
not create alternative solutions, but fosters a climate of creativity
in which staff members can design their own alternatives.

In summary, goal-oriented, process-centered, effective
nurse-managers will do the following:

- Encourage risk taking.
- Invest time.
- Eliminate noncontributing procedures.
- Guide problem solving.
- Aid in designing alternative solutions.

It goes without saying that when these tactics are tried, they often are met with negative vibrations. However, the nurse-manager can do at least five things to counteract any negative reaction:

1. *Be self-assured.* Effective nurse-managers remember who they are. They make it clear that they are self-confident and satisfied with their knowledge of how to accomplish things.
2. *Be influential.* Effective nurse-managers build a power base by either acquiring it or creating it. As they contribute to the organization, they are building power that can put them into increasingly higher circles of influence. When they seek opportunities to bring order out of chaos, they are practicing power relationships, which is just what they need.
3. *Be selective.* Effective nurse-managers choose the audience to hear their ideas. Because they are the ones guiding the decisions, they make sure that any contribution is most important for the interest of the hospital and patient care.
4. *Be cheerful.* Everybody gravitates toward the person who sees opportunities rather than problems. Everyone wants a better way, so effective nurse-managers talk about their vision of the better way or demonstrate a superior method.
5. *Be patient.* The way of management is not easy, so effective nurse-managers develop performance strategies that concentrate on several alternatives and options.

Armed with these *be*-attitudes, the nurse-manager can look forward to operating at full potential.

Peak Performance

Peak performer is a term used to describe a person who is operating at full potential. Peak performers are not superheroes. Rather, they are average persons who have fully developed their natural talents.

Peak performers have an action attitude that starts by self-movement. A prime attitude for the peak performer is a commitment to constructive discontent, a commitment to do things better. In a mental sense, managers who are peak performers ask themselves what they, not others, can do to be more effective, and they focus on the needed outcomes that will make a difference. Peak-performing nurse-managers dare to dream while their healthy discontent focuses on what can be. There is an attitude of "I can make a difference" and a sense of urgency.

When nurse-managers act as peak performers, they initiate interaction. This makes them proactive; they become their own choice-makers while assuming the responsibility for their own decisions. The hallmark of peak performers is the willingness to forego immediate gratification in order to gain greater reward later. Peak performers learn to say yes to their goals, keep their priorities, and say no to distractions. They are not afraid to have their ideas judged by others. The potential fulfilling nurse-manager creates a climate that supports risk taking because ideas, and often success, are generated by taking a calculated risk.

Peak performance does call for paying dues and a different mind-set of attitudes and self-perceptions, but a nurse-manager can practice at least 10 recognizable skills to improve performance:

1. *Develop a well-defined career path*. Peak performers know where they want to go in the corporate structures. They are persistent in making goals and in

developing strategies and tactics. Once a goal is accomplished, skills are upgraded.

2. *Develop good interpersonal skills.* With an ability to talk to anyone at any level in the organization, peak performers feel equally comfortable with the housekeeping staff or the CEO.

3. *Use resources.* Peak performers seek outside advice from experts without feeling insecure.

4. *Develop analytical skills.* Peak-performing nurse-managers take educated risks after analyzing the facts and weighing both sides of the issue.

5. *Develop written and oral communication skills.* Peak performers can express themselves without hesitation.

6. *Develop diversified outside interests.* The nurse-manager should not be restricted or confined to a narrow point of view.

7. *Differentiate a social network.* Business opportunities and business contacts are improved through peers and others.

8. *Be aware of company politics.* Peak performers find the best person to help push their ideas forward.

9. *Create an atmosphere of trust.* Problems can be solved when solutions are open for discussion.

10. *Visualize and use mental rehearsal.* A mental rehearsal of coming events gives an image of success.

These skills will be enhanced if the nurse-manager is aware that a peak performer can be characterized as a person who

- Has a singleness of purpose
- Is willing to devote enormous amounts of time and energy to achieve goals
- Has a stable personal life
- Enjoys challenges, decision making, and competition
- Rarely accepts defeat

To illustrate these peak-performance characteristics, consider this experience of a nurse-manager who heard that one of the ways the hospital could increase income was to do more outpatient business by being awarded the contract for care of senior citizens. By working long hours to determine the seniors' needs, exerting extra effort in determining the cost, developing a plan, and spending a lot of personal time tracking down the influential person who would award the contract, this manager was able to put the plan in action and thus increased outpatient volume.

If nurse-managers are serious about management and are willing to practice these performance-improvement skills and develop peak-performance characteristics, they have a good chance to operate at full potential.

Effectiveness Through Negotiation

Creating a climate of trust is one of the performance-improvement skills that should be mastered as soon as possible because it is the basis of negotiating behavior, an important management function. Trust determines the stance of willingness to negotiate. It can be defined as placing confidence, and it relies on truth and accuracy. To be successful at negotiating, the nurse-manager must be aware of the following:

- Staff members must feel there is no competition between themselves and the nurse-manager.
- The goals of the staff and the manager must not be totally divergent.
- Both staff and management operate within the basic framework of the same hospital climate and culture.

To create a climate that allows discussion, the nurse-manager does not show an open display of strength of position. Through discussion it may be possible to change the other person's mind, but *not* if the nurse-manager gives the idea that further discussion is closed.

To be successful, each negotiation builds on the last in terms of style and past performance. Each time the nurse-manager negotiates, the expectations and perceptions of staff members become more in tune with how the manager has reacted in the past. Allowing staff members to win concessions already decided upon by the manager gives control to both sides and allows for a win-win solution.

Good negotiators reveal their information in small pieces and ask many questions. The person who asks questions remains in control because asking questions forces the other side to give feedback and disclose information about its position. Sometimes, the use of a third-party case history may be valuable in letting the managment's position be known.

Delay is one of the best methods to use in negotiation. Delay does not give staff members an indication of the manager's intentions, but it does alter the situation dramatically in the manager's favor in case of a deadlock. Delay does not mean postponement. It means taking the time to develop the benefits of management's proposal and to determine flexible alternatives.[2] This bargaining process is a social exchange and is very important to the outcome of the negotiation.

To modify the ideas against management, the attitudes of staff members must be changed. Starting with preconceptions, existing beliefs, and needs, staff members must be moved towards the manager's proposition. When staff members agree, the manager provides immediate support. If staff members disagree, the manager provides gentle resistance or no support. Everyone involved in a bargaining situation tries to find a sense of balance between the two positions. Negotiation depends on both parties seeing a constructive solution to the problem at hand and a willingness to accept responsibility to change.

No matter how amiable the situation is, to maximize management's gain, to achieve the desired goal, the nurse-manager must change the perception of the staff. Three approaches may help change the staff's behavior and keep them from attacking a new idea:

1. Centering on the positive
2. Selling the idea on the basis of its merit
3. Being enthusiastic about the new options

Consider this example: Recently, when a medical unit was restructured so that all the respiratory-bound patients could be placed in a special section, the nurse-manager really believed that this was a good move that would improve the quality and provide more cost-effective care. She tried to keep the reason for change staff-centered by pointing out to staff members how the clustering of the patients in one area would cut down on the time spent in approaching the patients and in gathering the needed supplies. Furthermore, not only the nurses but the respiratory technicians would find that access to one type of patient would save time and effort.

It is important to strengthen the argument for staff members as to how they will benefit because it will strengthen the principle of mutual gain. If staff members firmly resist change, it is tempting to defend, criticize, or reject their ideas. However, with both sides defending their own ideas, the direction of negotiation slips to defending personalities. If the staff members push, the nurse-manager must not push back but must break the cycle by not reacting to anger. It is better to diffuse the staff members' anger by acknowledging their tactics used to dissuade.

Staff members will use three tactics to dissuade the manager:

1. Pushing their position to extremes
2. Attacking management's position
3. Attacking management personally

To combat these tactics, the nurse-manager must look behind the staff to define the staff's position and what caused it.

A good negotiator will use the staff members' position as an alternative solution and refine it. Eliminating the personalities from the discussion, and then raising questions about management's position will diffuse the issue.

When the nurse-manager in the previous example presented the change involving the respiratory unit, staff members pointed out that their job descriptions did not limit them to respiratory care. They attacked the manager's position as being one designed only to cut costs without thought of quality and then blamed the whole move on the nurse-manager's dislike of respiratory patients. In the staff meeting the nurse-manager acknowledged that cost was the issue and emphasized all the factors that would enhance the quality of care.

Should nurse-managers find themselves up against a more powerful opponent, a situation in which negotiations probably will not come to a close, a scenario for options should be developed. This is the time for finding the best alternative and providing a practical option. While trying to develop this alternative, it is necessary to try to anticipate the last alternative of the opponent. All negotiators must remember that a successful negotiation may entail *not* coming to the original goal.

For example, not too long ago a physician requested that his patient receive extensive diabetic teaching from the nurse-educator. The nurse-manager could not fulfill his request because that position had been rescinded by recent budget cuts, but she offered to have one of the staff nurses start the diabetic teaching. The physician countered by asking that the teaching be done on an outpatient basis. This was a successful negotiation in which neither party came to the original goal.

Bargainers work together in search of mutual goals. Research on negotiation has shown that matching strategies elicits a positive response from the other party.[2] Matching gives the staff members the perception that the nurse-manager is both firm and fair. In other words, the nurse-manager must concede an argument every time the staff concedes an argument.

In summary, these are the points to remember about negotiation:

1. Each negotiation builds on the last.
2. Information should be revealed in small pieces.
3. Delay is a good negotiation tactic.
4. Negotiation depends on changing attitudes.
5. Negotiation depends on changing perceptions.
6. Arguments about the staff's gain should be strengthened.
7. The staff's position for disagreement should be defined.
8. A scenario for options should be developed.
9. Strategies should be matched.

Leadership as a Function of Management

As much as negotiating is a function of management, so is leadership. Leadership is an action that involves the activities of persuasion, invitation, argument, publicity, dependence on the logic of events, a demonstration of affectionate devotion, and the provision for typical problem situations for enhancing learning in organizations.[3] Leadership is an interpersonal influence, exercised in situations and directed through communication toward the attainment of specific goals. It has been suggested that leadership cannot be taught or learned, that it is obtained from the social environment and from learning.

Confusion exists about the terms leader and manager because persons who are leaders are rarely perceived as such until they exhibit leadership within a group. This makes it difficult to distinguish between the process of management and the function of leadership. As pointed out before, a manager is one who is responsible for achieving results through others. A leader, on the other hand, is one who delegates by availability. A leader can be described as transactional, one who trades one commodity for another. Additionally, leaders can be transforming. The transforming leader defines an existing need of a follower, matches it with an organization's goal, and then promotes it.[4] Transformational leaders produce social change that satisfies followers' needs.

Leadership takes on aspects that involve subordinates in decisions. When decisions are delegated, independence is fostered. A leader uses persuasion and shares power and responsibility with staff members. The leader must use power effectively. This includes enlisting cooperation. As long as the leader is able to keep the activity staff-centered, the result will be participation.

Leaders, such as nurse-managers, serve two masters. They serve the hospital organization, and they serve the staff they manage. That is to say, the hospital expects high levels of productivity from the nurse-manager, and staff members expect personal need-satisfying rewards from the nurse-manager. This requires that the nurse-manager become an exchange agent by trying to encourage staff members to increase their productivity while trying to improve the quality of their work life. One step that a leader can take is to delegate some of the responsibility to the staff. This helps staff members ensure their output and gives them some control over their own destinies.

Certain leadership functions can be shared with group members; others can be performed only by the leader. In a hospital, for example, the nurse-manager is the person who has primary responsibility for linking the work group to the rest of the hospital. The leader has full responsibility for the staff's performance and for seeing that staff members meet the demands and expectations placed on them by the rest of the organization of which they are a part. Other members of the staff may share this responsibility at times, but the leader never can avoid full responsibility for adequate performance of the group.

Although the leader accepts the responsibility and influence of the organization, there is a concerted effort to de-emphasize status. This can be accomplished by doing the following:

- Listening well and patiently
- Not being impatient with the progress of the group, particularity on difficult problems
- Accepting more blame than may be warranted for any failure or mistake
- Giving the group members ample opportunity to express their thoughts
- Being careful never to impose a decision upon a group
- Putting personal contributions in the forms of questions or stating them speculatively
- Arranging for others to perform leadership functions that enhance their status

To illustrate, a nurse-manager observed the ED staff members doing an excellent job of taking care of several trauma cases over a short period of time. She observed that the staff had developed two routines that cut through the standard procedures. During a staff meeting as a follow-up of this event, the nurse-manager listened to the group discuss the shortened routines. Putting her management status aside, she listened as a *fellow worker* and recognized that these routines not only were more efficient than the old procedure but also assured quality of care.

It is up to the leader to strengthen the group processes by seeing that all problems that involve the staff are dealt with by the staff. A leader never handles such problems outside the group, nor with individual members of the group. Although the leader is careful to see that all matters that affect and involve the whole group are handled by the whole group, the leader is equally alert not to undertake in a group meeting agenda items or tasks that do not concern the group. Matters concerning one individual member and only that member are, of course, handled individually. Matters involving only a subgroup are handled by that subgroup. The total group is kept informed, however, of any subgroup action.

The nurse-manager, as leader, fully reflects and effectively represents the views, goals, values, and decisions of the staff members to other hospital groups. In this way leadership is providing communication and exercising influence in both directions. Here are some other leadership skills:

- Adequate competence to handle the technical problems faced by the staff or provision for access to this technical knowledge
- Group-centeredness
- Ability to discourage complacency and passive acceptance of the present
- Ability to be enthusiastic about the mission and goals of the organization
- Sensitive supportive relationships

These are the skills that can improve the leadership function of nurse-managers, thus enabling them to have an enormous impact on the growth and development of their staff members.

Conflict Resolution

Conflict is a competitive or opposing action of incompatibles, an antagonistic state with divergent ideas, or mental struggles resulting from incompatible external or internal demands. Conflict is not only unavoidable but also essential to the growth of any organism or any organization. It is the management of conflict that comes under scrutiny. Conflict management should have as its goal neither suppression nor elimination of conflict but, instead, resolution of conflict. More specifically, the manager's handling of conflict among subordinates must be done in a way that will enhance the goals of both the individual and the organization.

In wise conflict management, actions or inactions, escalation or withdrawal, that can lead to destructive forces should be avoided. It is important to know when to intervene and when not to.

Successful management of conflict toward productive, goal-enhancing resolution demands that management understand both the intrapersonal and the interpersonal dynamics of conflict. Even more important is a correct determination of the sources of conflict.

Likert and Likert[5] suggested that there are two basic kinds of conflict: substantive and affective. That is, conflict is a part of organization life, or it relates to or arises from feelings and emotions of the members of the organization.

More specifically, conflict can be caused by the denial of basic human rights to determine one's own destiny. A second source of personal conflict occurs as the result of the "changingness" of the organization as it responds to environmental demands. If individual employees attempt to maintain the status quo, or if they experience a loss of self-esteem because of changing roles and obsolescence of their jobs, tension erupts into conflict. A third cause occurs as a result when persons who interact overestimate the importance of their own positions and underestimate the importance of the others' positions.

Sometimes it is the system itself that promotes conflict. Katz et al[6] noted that one of the problems in human relations occurs as a result of differences in perception, of two or more persons viewing the same situation in different ways. However, differences in perception are not sufficient reason for conflict. It is perceptions distorted by individual values, expectations, and needs that cause a transition from differing to conflict.

For instance, recently a hospital had to take drastic measures for cutting its budget. A management analyst had said that the nursing units had too many layers of management. Following suggestions to trim, some supervisory positions were eliminated. Nurses holding those positions were offered the position of staff nurse. When the former supervisors assumed the positions of staff nurses, the other staff nurses perceived the reason as demotion and in conflict with supervisory status.

The most "malignant" kind of conflict among subordinates is generated by an insecure manager who unconsciously fears that a cohesive group would usurp power or, in their strength, expose weaknesses.[7] Such a manager encourages dissident groups among subordinates by arbitrarily giving and withholding rewards and by faulty or selective communication.

Another primary factor in conflict is egoistic communication. This includes assuming that others understand what has been said or that the listeners, in turn, understand what has not been said. Accustomed to using words such as productivity, cost containment, and downsizing, the nurse-manager easily can exclude staff participation. Management language can turn off staff members. When these management-centered terms must be used, they must be defined and clarified with examples.

Another source of conflict is just being in a group activity because group activity involves choice and decision making.[8] Decision making can cause tension because choosing alternatives includes a loss-gain factor and a requirement to "live with" decisions after they are made.

Conflict also can occur as a result of time lag, lack of feedback, diffusion of control, technical obsolescence, or the failure to strike a balance between the independent and dependent needs of the staff members.

The point to remember is that without conflict goals would not be achieved, and problems would not get solved. Other positive outcomes of conflict include an expanded understanding of more effective ways of dealing with the issues. Resources and energies are mobilized and heightened in the process of confronting and dealing with conflicts, and creative searching for alternatives and solutions enhances the ability of subordinates to work together in the future.[9]

The nurse-manager plays a vital role in conflict resolution. The necessity and inevitability of conflicts in an organization demand that relevant skills be mastered. Effective conflict resolution requires an understanding of self and of personal values, goals, and inner conflicts and the ability to see the various components of a conflict situation as a whole.[10]

The ideal conflict resolution is designed by the organization that encourages communications as ongoing fact gathering in a positive atmosphere that treats conflict as a constructive occurrence. Conflict resolution requires action, either by the employee or by the organization itself. Strategies for managing conflict are seldom easy or simple. Major, lasting changes in serious conflict problems usually involve ongoing and extensive efforts by managers to remove the obstacles. Main[2] described four major obstacles to conflict resolution:

1. *Selective perception*. Persons see *and* hear what is expected.
2. *Passing judgment*. Persons evaluate what is seen and heard, rather than listening to what is seen and heard.
3. *Lack of facts*. Resolution depends on *all* the facts.
4. *Cloudy thinking*. Dichotomizing a situation in the extreme makes it either win or lose.

Likert[11] suggested that conflict resolution is only possible if it can be converted from a win-lose negotiation to a problem-solving situation. In this way all parties can emerge as winners. It is necessary to first differentiate between what is essential in the outcomes and what would be desirable. It must be stressed that conflict management is resolution seeking, not argument winning.

Nurse-managers must honor at least seven major rules in conflict resolution to keep conflict constructive and healthy[7]:

1. Ensure effective communication networks and practices.
2. Manage the relationships between parties so that some do not emerge as perceived losers.
3. Avoid compromise as a solution.
4. When at all possible, seek to head off destructive conflict.

5. Act as chief pacifier of destructive conflict.
6. Remain problem-centered rather than personality-centered.
7. Structure the organization so that destructive conflict does not occur.

When these rules are honored, and energy is focused on overall goals of the organization, effective ongoing procedures for conflict intervention will emerge. Four different classes of conflict intervention exist[9]:

1. Redirecting immediate behavior
2. Reallocating relevant resources
3. Reframing perspectives of the conflict
4. Realigning structural forces that underlie the situation

Redirecting behavior is essential when too much conflict may have produced deadlocks and when the acceptable alternatives have become restricted to two incompatible positions. Interventions that offer previously unrecognized alternatives may help unfreeze parties who otherwise could not abandon their commitments or views. For example, not too long ago, the laundry in a nearby hospital decided to change laundry hampers to increase production and lower costs. When the nurses were informed of the impending change, they stormed the material manager's office. They declared that they would not use the proposed hampers. Needless to say, the laundry management and the nurses were at a deadlock. At that point, delegates from nursing and the laundry management looked over many types of laundry hampers before finding a third type of hamper that satisfied everyone.

When too little conflict exists, when suppression or withdrawal from the controversy has failed to produce any alternatives, then interventions that focus on "hard choices" or on "trade-offs" may expand the vision of the contestants.

In both types of conflict, too much or too little, communication usually has stopped. Strategies that encourage the sharing of perceptions are often effective at unblocking communication. When conflict has escalated, the most effective tactic for creating cooperation from conflict is to use a nonpunitive response that combines some self-defense for both parties with a willingness to cooperate. When too little conflict exists, important issues will not surface or be resolved. In the initial intervention, it is important that managers establish the attitude that avoidance of differences is inconsistent with the organizational climate.

Another effective intervention is reallocating resources. With this intervention management can either expand or diminish the available personnel, information, or other resources relevant to the conflict. This might mean redesigning productivity schedules or requirements.

The fourth type of conflict intervention, realigning underlying forces, can be accomplished by altering the situational conditions that generate conflict. Examples are including new members in the group, making more relevant information available, or renegotiating norms and values.

This brings to mind the conflict between nurses and respiratory technicians. Even though the hospital sees a need for the technician, the nurse in the intensive care unit (ICU) wants to have complete charge of the patient care. The nurse and the technician can lock horns, or the nurse-manager can step in, have a team meeting, explain cost-effective quality of care, and point out their common goals.

Clearly, the interventions for conflict, not the elimination of conflict, must be emphasized. Equally clear is the fact that conflict is a part of organizational life. Conflict includes interpersonel, intrapersonal, situational, and organizational dimensions and, as a highly complex phenomenon, has the potential to either enhance or destroy.

Whenever possible, and when the nature of the organization permits it, an interaction-influence network is the best strategy for managing conflict. This is a design that encourages greater utilization of the human potential and minimizes or eliminates destructive conflict.

Individuality is not only respected but valued. Such organizations also seem to be able to manage conflict because their primary focus is on building effective work groups with high performance goals.

In summary, to be effective, nurse-managers must dare to take risks, operate at full potential, create a climate of trust for negotiation, lead subordinates toward decisions, and recognize conflict as essential to the growth of the organization.

The next chapter discusses how all of these management functions can be enhanced by skillful communication.

References

1. Drucker PF: *Management*. New York, Harper & Row Publishers Inc, 1973.
2. Main J: How to be a better negotiator. *Fortune*, September 1983.
3. Tead O: *The Art of Administration*. New York, McGraw-Hill Book Co, 1951.
4. Burns JM: *Conflict as an Opportunity to Display Leadership*. New York, Harper & Row Publishers Inc, 1978.
5. Likert R, Likert JG: *New Ways of Managing Conflict*. New York, McGraw-Hill Book Co, 1976.
6. Katz RL, Wolfe DM, Quinn EP, et al: Human relations skills can be sharpened. *Harvard Bus Rev*, July/August 1956, p 61.
7. Odiorne G: *Personnel Administration by Objectives*. Howard, Ill, Richard D Irwin Inc, 1971.
8. Napier R: *Groups: Theories and Experience*. Boston, Houghton Mifflin Co, 1973.
9. Brown LD: *Managing Conflict at Organizational Interfaces*. Menlo Park, Calif, Addison-Wesley Publishing Co Inc, 1983.
10. Katz RL: Skills of an effective administrator. *Harvard Bus Rev*, September/October 1974, p 90.
11. Likert R: A method for coping with conflict in problem-solving groups. *Group Org Stud* 1978.

Chapter 4

Communication: The Nerve Center of Management

Communication is comparable to the nervous system of the human body. The very life of a nursing division depends on communication, and failure to communicate is a symptom of organizational neuropathy. The nerves of the organization literally can become atrophied or severed, permitting a minimal flow of information through the channels. There are many reasons why these "wires" can lose their ability to send and receive messages. Often it is an inability of the nurse-manager to tell staff members what they are to observe and listen for or what information should be transmitted upward.

Communication in management depends on sensors. These sensors, which are analogous to nerve tips, permeate each management division. They must sense and sort all the vital information from all the nursing shifts. This information is the very life stimulus for decision making and depends on an informed staff. When different individuals throughout the division are groomed and trained in the art of listening and communicating, they will act as sensors, and the probability of keeping in touch with vital information about patients, politics, and performances will be higher. Communication is an important function of the nurse-manager.

Nurse-managers are prime agents for both intragroup and intergroup communication. They are the main channel for communicating the effectiveness of their group. It is their responsibility to gain recognition and stature for their staff and, particularly, for high-producing individuals.

A nurse-manager has a responsibility to communicate downward, but a greater emphasis is on communicating the unit's accomplishments to higher management to gain influence for the unit. Many a nursing unit has found itself in a state of mere existence, with no one paying attention to it. This unit seems to function by itself in an isolated corner. Sometimes such units are the subject of inquiry. People begin to ask, "What does that unit do?" This is an example of how the nurse-manager has failed in the responsibility of transmission, an important phase of the communication process.

Employees look to the nurse-manager to transmit information that represents their accomplishments. Employees churn emotionally because their nurse-manager has not focused attention on their contribution. Many nursing units fail to get their budget requests approved because a nurse-manager has not relayed staff-defined fiscal needs. Because top management has not been informed, budget allocations are limited. An effective nurse-manager will transmit the group's accomplishments not only to have the high-achieving individuals identified but also to have top management recognize a manager with communication skills.

What Needs to be Communicated?

Even though nurse-managers must communicate the facts about patient goals and service purposes of their units, it is important that they communicate feelings also. Sometimes top management forgets what a certain unit is doing. Somehow the output and the "hands-on" mission are lost. This may cause the staff members to become restless, unhappy, and dissatisfied. At other times staff members may be happy and chomping at the bit with enthusiasm because their efforts have been recognized. These different feeling states must be transmitted to top management to keep them informed of the working climate.

Nurse-managers communicate needs and problems for performance effectiveness. Nurse-managers who state that everything is running smoothly are deceiving themselves and misleading top management. They must focus not only on problems but also on the barriers to accomplishing the projected objectives of their units.

This does not suggest that nurse-managers should be "rebels without a cause," rather they should be "communicators with a cause." When there are feelings and problems that could cause barriers to success, the nurse-manager must communicate them. Top management cannot help the nurse-manager unless the intimate details about feelings and problems have been communicated.

What Do Staff Members Want to Know?

Staff members should have a broad overview of patient and political activities. They are interested in knowing the financial impact of their activities on the total health care system. They also want to know what higher management needs. It is up to the nurse-manager to tell them what is true and what is not true.

Rumors are the first hint of topside problems, so it is up to the nurse-manager to communicate the exact nature of any problem in the hospital. Given the truth and the opportunity, staff members will come up with suggestions to correct the problems. This will give them an opportunity to identify with the welfare of the hospital. Sharing in problem solving results in increased group cohesiveness and solidification.

The Process of Communication

Communication involves three stages: (1) the production of

the message, (2) the transmission of the message, and (3) the reception of the message. As a sender of messages, the nurse-manager needs to improve skills in making, transmitting, and receiving messages to establish more effective relationships.

Communication is an understanding process. As the sender, the nurse-manager must plan the intent of what is sent and the response desired. This requires an understanding of the signals and cues that are transmitted with the message.

The purpose of communication is threefold: (1) to impart or give information so the receiver can respond to the message sent (the intended message), (2) to get feedback about how the message is being received, and (3) to send signals that indicate an interest in building and sustaining an interpersonal relationship.

Communication is the means by which interests can be shared with other staff members while building a relationship. This sharing can be viewed as an interpersonal acceptance and awareness of one another's humanness—a process that includes the following:

- *Dealing with complexity*. Everyone has repressed desires, memories, and hidden needs that influence the personality. The complexity of personality begins with the self and extends to others whom a person meets and works with to achieve certain goals. Each person feels or senses the impact of another's complexity. As a result, everyone needs to strive for open communication. Comprehension of the self in relationship to these interpersonal complexities results in a better understanding of personhood.

- *Decreasing anxiety*. Anxiety can be decreased through sharing, which increases predictability in relationships. Unpredictability can be so great that persons sometimes put on "role masks" and resort to cliches and gamesmanship. The purpose of sharing, or communicating about the self, is to create a predictable structure, a relationship through which messages can and will be accepted emotionally. This interchange increases predictability and helps reduce any feelings of threat.

- *Dialogue*. Dialogue is open talking through which things are shared in terms of what is important to both persons. A certain amount of superficial chatter can be endured, but each person has a need, a desire, to understand and present a view of those things that have a deeper meaning. Dialogue is authentic and creative when ideas are exchanged that can lead to personal growth.

- *Dynamics*. Dynamics involves a sincere interest that stimulates and sustains an ongoing relationship. As persons spend the day talking to colleagues, they soon find that they enjoy the healthy, free-flowing exchange of thoughts and sincere exchange of ideas. This marks the pattern of growth for the involved individuals.

- *The Context of the Message*. The choice of words tells a great deal about a person. The ways that words are expressed throw light on the meaning of the message. The clarity of the message depends largely on the precise use of words, simple exact language, and good grammar. Even facial gestures, hand signals, and other body language are related to the way a message is received and interpreted.

Avoiding Communication Blocks

Messages must be aimed at a level that the receiver will understand. The nurse-manager should not talk down to the receivers or over their heads. If the nurse-manager senses that a listener does not understand what is being said, the manager should not be afraid to say politely, "Tell me, please, what you just heard me say." When talking with others, the nurse-manager should be careful not to assume that they have the comprehension level that the manager expects them to have. There is not necessarily a high correlation between education and communication comprehension.

Other blocks to communication include speaking too rapidly, high anxiety in the listener, distracting nervous gestures, and group interference. These can be avoided if speakers do the following:

1. Remain aware of how fast they are talking. (Does the speaker understand what is being said?)
2. Test the anxiety level in the audience. (Is the audience apprehensive or uneasy?)
3. Remain aware of any personal nervous gestures. (These include clearing the throat, facial twitches, and shaky hands.)
4. Choose the place for sending the message. (Personal messages should not be delivered in front of a group.)

The best way to avoid blocks to communication is to anticipate them and prevent them.

The Timing of Communication

The timing of any message is important. Even though the message may be precise, it can be ineffective if the timing is wrong. To select the right moment for maximum effect for getting the message across, it is necessary to study the situation. The listener cannot be preoccupied with other things. There must be enough allotted time available so that all of the message can be transmitted.

The Impact of Communication

An awareness of the impact of the message on the receiver is important. Effective communication requires a sensitivity in knowing as much about the other person as possible. This capacity for participating in another's feelings is called empathy. It is through this profound and somewhat mysterious process that understanding, influence, and significant relationships between persons take place. The more one person can climb into the skin of another in terms of who the other is as a person, the more the first person can understand the other's world and the way the other functions. This is what it takes for interpersonal linkage and communication bonding.

Receiving and Sending Messages

One function of the nurse-manager is to interpret and amplify the received signals. Some are explicit verbal signals; others are more covert cues that require actual reading. Awareness of nonverbal cues can help a person communicate and ascertain whether and how the communication has been received.

It is not always what is said, but how it is said, that makes the difference. Variance in voice tone can give the phrase "thanks a lot" totally different meanings. Words are interpreted in terms of personal experience. The message is in the ear of the receiver, not the sender. A blank stare or a quizzical expression indicates that the message is not understood. That is why phrases such as these are heard: "What I mean to say is...," or "By that I mean...."

The nurse-manager should be alert to and respond to the barriers of communication by developing some of these different strategies:

- *Being creatively aware.* This involves adopting an attitude that effective communication is a mission possible rather than a mission impossible. The nurse-manager is aware that a relationship can mean that two persons can become aware of each other's needs and make choices together. The listener does not feel threatened when the sender senses the possibility of working creatively together.

- *Avoiding the position of confrontation*. When the position of confrontation is assumed, the silent message is, "I am going to take you on . . . . it's my will against yours." If this is the message that is received, then anxiety is increased. With high levels of anxiety any proposal of working creatively together will not be heard. Any words sent from a position of confrontation will be interpreted as an invitation for conflict and challenge. The result is that productivity may deteriorate into interpersonal friction and fault finding.

- *Avoiding control and competition words*. The listener may accurately (or inaccurately) receive and decode the message as an indication of a desire for control, competition, domination, and power, situations that are disliked in an interpersonal interaction. The reaction would be to fight or flee.

- *Conveying collaboration*. The receiver needs to get the message in both a context and a content that imply a recognition of the need for mutual change. It is imperative to send a message that tells about similar interests, questions, and information, a message that will indicate the possibility of cooperation for mutual gain. In effect that message says, "We don't have to be afraid of each another."

- *Identify commonality*. When a message that suggests a desire to start, build, and sustain a relationship is heard as only a weak signal, the receiver will approach the new relationship cautiously. The communicating nurse-manager will convey the needs and ideas held in common and stress the need for association to accomplish common goals.

In other words, a message that is conveyed with personal excitement increases effectiveness. When many things are going on around a person, interest is not aroused easily. However, if the message appeals to the needs and motivations that the receiver has at that time, the message will be heard. Nurse-managers need to package the content of their communication in terms of personal appeal to gain the greatest attention.

Organizational Communication

Every step in the operation of an organization is dependent on communication.[1] Communication provides members with shared knowledge about an organization's goals, it is the vehicle by which an organization is embedded in its culture, and it transmits the inputs and outputs of an organization.

From a management's standpoint, an organization is an elaborate set of interconnected communication channels designed to collect, analyze, and sort information. These channels provide a means for making decisions, executing them, obtaining feedback, and correcting objectives and procedures. Organized activity ceases to exist and individual uncoordinated activity returns when communication stops.

Communication can be restricted by the structure of the organization. Formal structure often is inferred by the organizational chart and defined in terms of formal relationships and duties, job descriptions, rules, operating policies, work procedures, and arrangements for compensation.

By knowing the formal structure of the organization as displayed in the organizational chart, the type of information flow can be predicted. For example, in a hierarchy the information flow is vertical and more often downward. In a matrix the information flow is often horizontal and more often upward.

Horizontal flow of information is more frequent than vertical flow because individuals communicate more openly and effectively with their peers than with superiors. Horizontal exchanges are less subject to distortion because partners and peers share a common frame of reference. Furthermore, the contents of the messages carried by horizontal flow concern task-coordinated information, whereas those carried by downward flow are mainly authoritative, and those carried by upward flow provide feedback on performance. This means that the vertical messages are potentially more threatening, whereas the horizontal messages are more informal.

Beneath this formal structure is a more complex system of social relationships that form the structure of the informal networks. This informal structure is the breeding place of rumors. These unconfirmed messages, often lacking evidence, are transmitted by face-to-face channels. They may be inaccurate, but they often convey some truth. It is the wise manager who taps the grapevine to get to the real feelings of the employees about a proposed change.

When it comes to change, two-way trust in all matters, especially communication, must be conveyed and emphasized. Communications are better in high-trust situations. Individuals who trust one another may not communicate accurately, but this is not necessarily an impediment to getting something done. Because they trust, they feel that it is not absolutely necessary to figure out precisely what the other is trying to say. Openness and trust in the change process therefore influence whether and how change occurs.[2]

Many changes in a hospital are brought about by changes in the hospital culture. Consequently, for any hospital to be innovative, it must demonstrate openness, a receptivity to the exchange of information with its people. Upward, negative feedback is also important for change because change depends on accurate accounts of the actual accomplishments at the bottom of the organization. In other words, the rate of change depends on open communication and on adequate communication channels for upward flow of negative feedback.

Could there be a strong relationship between the directional flow of communication and job satisfaction of hospital professionals?[6] Is it possible that nurses react more positively (are more satisfied) when the information flow is in all directions (ie, up, down, and between peers)? This suggests that even though a formal structure is used by administrative personnel, a more flexible hospital culture that provides open and free-flowing information may be necessary for nurses.[3]

As the values of the hospital culture gradually changed to include cost-effectiveness with the passion for caring for humankind, businesses became partners with the nurses, and a subtle change in communication took place. Too often it was dismissed as failure in communications, but it goes deeper than that. Most business terminology is masculine and almost a foreign speech to women. It is replete with secret codes, double meanings, and colloquial slang. It falls into three general subject categories: military derivations, sports lingo, and sexual allusions.[4] Nurse-managers must learn to translate this jargon correctly, or they will miss the deeper meaning and true significance of what is being said to them, about them, or around them. Because the value of understanding a language but pretending not to is a shrewd political move, it is strongly recommended that each nurse-manager read Harragan's ideas about business jargon.[4]

Applying These Communication Strategies

In the bustling world of the hospital, how can nurse-managers be sure that everybody gets the message? Wlody[5] has designed a five-step approach:

Step 1. Sharpen personal communication techniques.
- Be sure to use precise, clear terms.
- Include all essential information.
- Let voice and manner convey positive messages.
- Convey a democratic leadership style.

Step 2. Assist the staff in developing the skill of communication.
- Identify the types of problems that develop from communication breakdowns.

- Get staff to identify positive and negative types of communication and give examples.
- Record and share observed examples of communication.
- Suggest ways to improve communication in future transactions.

Step 3. Lead the staff into more positive interactions.

- Create a democratic environment in which more staff members can participate.
- Hold staff meetings to share positive and negative events.

Step 4. Make daily rounds with the whole team.

- Explore shared concerns about patient care.
- Initiate multidisciplinary rounds in order to *exchange* ideas, not to report to each other.
- Shared planning allows greater input by the nurses whose status can become higher because of presentation of vital information.

Step 5. Form a group to reduce stress.

- Mutual sharing of problems and solutions strengthens communication networks.

Establishing sound communication within the hospital is a real challenge to nurse-managers. Developing a sharp personal communication style is very important, but it is only half the job. The nurse-manager must convince staff members that communication is a necessary skill that augments other patient-care practices.

Finally, communication in the hospital deals with accomplishing tasks and adjusting social, emotional, or employment issues. It is essential in defining job performance and maintaining productivity. Honest communication offers the key to finding out why and how a staff is motivated.

References

1. Rogers EM, Agarwala-Rogers R: Organizational communication, in Hanneman GJ, McEwan WJ (eds): *Communication and Behavior*. Menlo Park, Calif, Addison-Wesley Publishing Co Inc, 1975.
2. Deal TE, Kennedy AA: *Corporate Cultures*. Menlo Park, Calif, Addison-Wesley Publishing Co Inc, 1982.
3. Applebaum SH: *Stress Management for Health Care Professionals*. Rockville Md, Aspen Systems Corp, 1981.
4. Harragan BL: *Games Mother Never Taught You*. Warner Books, 1977.
5. Wlody GS: Communicating in the ICU: Do you read me loud and clear? *Nurs Management*, September 1984, pp 24-29.

Chapter 5

Managing Motivation

During the 1980s improving performance in hospitals will be related directly to how well personnel are motivated through meaningful work. This motivation requires the application of behavior science theory and practice. Hospitals have responded in various ways. Many have offered better pay and job security to nurses only to find that the response has been discouraging.

Hospital consultants have heard many nurses express dissatisfactions about their nursing jobs and have watched nurses leave a profession at an annual turnover rate of 37% to 67%.[1] Nurses who are not leaving appear to be seriously evaluating the costs and benefits associated with joining unions.[2] It seems that young nurses who have been reared in an affluent society find little value in holding jobs that they consider menial or nonchallenging. Although younger nurses are probably as committed as older nurses to their work, they are demanding greater job satisfaction. They want their jobs to be interesting and challenging, and they want to participate more in shaping their work environment. This presents a problem because these humanistic expectations and demands are at odds with work conditions and managerial practices of many hospitals.[3]

Some hospitals have concluded that the job, not the nurse, must be changed and have introduced some changes in job content and managerial practices. Others have delegated more authority and responsibility to the staff and permitted them to participate in decision making. These different practices share an underlying theme that the survival of a hospital depends on the attainment of both individual and hospital goals.

Attainment of individual and organizational goals is mutually interdependent and linked by a common denominator—employee motivation.[3] Nurses are motivated to satisfy their personal goals, and they should be able to contribute their efforts to the attainment of hospital goals as a means of achieving their personal goals. Motivation, therefore, can be considered the key to individual well-being and organizational success.

The Nature of Motivation

Motivation refers to goal-directed behavior that is influenced not only by the individual's needs, interests, attitudes, and goals but also by the tasks, managerial practices, and climate of the organization.[3] Motivation is also a performance commitment that results from the employee's inner needs to work because of the intrinsic meaningfulness of the job.[4]

Understanding how a person's needs are manifested into goal-directed behavior is the first step in studying motivational behavior. A need is an internal state of disequilibrium that causes a person to pursue certain courses of action to regain equilibrium. Every person has a set of needs, and satisfying these needs becomes the goal of self-directed behavior.

Nurses are often attracted to a certain hospital because that hospital can provide them with various means of satisfying their needs. Existence needs, for example, can be met with pay. Affiliation needs can be met with opportunities for socializing and participating. Personal development needs can be met by working in a creative climate. Attractive salaries, socialization opportunities, and a chance for creativity are ways to encourage people to join an organization and are called incentives.

Interaction of these incentives, perceptual patterns of the individual, and personal needs brings about motivation. That is, a person's needs push for a certain action for satisfaction, whereas incentives pull that person toward a certain organization.

Nurse-managers cannot influence staff behavior unless they understand the nature of the needs that motivate each staff member. Because staff members have different needs and to different degrees, they will respond to the same organizational incentives in different ways. Therefore, to influence the behavior of each staff member in a desired direction, the nurse-manager must actually assess each member's needs.

Maslow[5] viewed an individual's motivation in terms of a needs hierarchy arranged in the order of the intensity of the underlying drives:

1. Physiologic
2. Safety
3. Social
4. Self-esteem
5. Self-actualization

Physiologic needs are those associated with hunger, thirst, rest, sex, and other biologic needs. Safety needs are needs for protection from danger, threat, and deprivation. Social needs are needs for expression of love and friendship. Self-esteem needs are composed of autonomy, dignity, and respect for others. Self-actualization needs are the needs for realizing one's own potentialities in the forms of creativity and the capacity for continuous self-development.

Each person, then, as a needy creature, rarely reaches a state of complete satisfaction and therefore continuously searches for satisfaction of personal needs. As soon as the needs on the lower level are reasonably satisfied, those on the next higher level will emerge as the dominant needs demanding satisfaction. According to Maslow,[5] a satisfied need is no longer a motivation for behavior. Deprivation, however, can be a motivator. It must be emphasized that needs rarely are found in isolation but instead in a variety of combinations. A certain behavior can be caused not by one need but by many needs. Also, an action can satisfy not one need but a whole set of needs.

Motivators and Dissatisfiers

Although this needs hierarchy may provide a key to motivation, it leaves questions to be answered. Herzberg[6] suggested that lower-order needs never get satisfied. This is shown by the constant demand for physiologic and security guarantees, the continuing socialization, and the never ending search for status symbols. He contends that two separate sets of needs are involved: The first is the built-in drive to avoid pain from the environment (eg, hunger), which drives a person to earn money. The second is the need for psychologic growth, which drives the individual to achieve. In the work setting, psychologic growth needs, the motivators, are met by job content, and pain avoidance needs, the dissatisfaction avoidance needs, are met by the job environment.

Factors that can bring on dissatisfaction are found in company policy and administration, supervisors, interpersonal relationships, working conditions, salary, status, and security. Factors that can bring about psychologic growth are found in achievement, the work itself, creativity, responsibility, and advancement.

Motivators and dissatisfiers reflect a two-dimensional needs structure: one system for the avoidance of dissatisfaction and a parallel system for personal growth (Table 5-1). Therefore, a healthy environment tries to prevent discontent with a job and offers opportunities for self-realization.

One observation cannot be overlooked at this point: It is not possible to motivate anyone to perform well who does not have the ability to do so. A person must have the requisite skills before that person can perform. However, many persons are more willing to suggest that they are not being motivated than to admit that they cannot do something. Employees can use motivation as a smoke screen to hide behind. Training, therefore, is often necessary, and it can itself be a powerful motivator.

The concern is how to motivate employees, not just move them. The main distinction between movement and motivation is duration. Moved workers do not get far before they must be moved again, whereas motivated workers move much further under their own initiative. Movement is a function of extrinsic fear and extrinsic reward. Motivation is a function of ability over potential, or opportunity over ability.[6]

Job Enrichment

One way to ensure good work performance is job enrichment. Herzberg[7] proposed that at least eight ingredients should be considered in the job-enrichment process.

1. *Direct feedback*. Knowing the results of one's behavior is essential to efficient learning and performance. The results of a person's performance should be given directly to the individual rather than through a supervisor.
2. *Client relationship*. Employees should recognize that they have customers to serve rather than just employers.
3. *Learning function*. All jobs should provide an opportunity for learning or outside training as a way of personal growth.
4. *The right to schedule their own work*. The staff persons who do the job are generally the most aware of the time available to spend on various aspects of the work. Allowing them to schedule their own work will make them responsible for the work—not responsible *to* the schedule.
5. *Control over their own resources*. Let the job holders have their own budgets, and let them manage those budgets for their operations. With expense accounts or approved budgets, they themselves will control the expenditures.

6. *Direct communication.* All employees should be able to communicate directly with each other and not be blocked by organizational lines. Too often the organizational chart represents the lines of communication, which causes overcommunication, and important things are lost. Direct communication makes it possible to be active and selective, with the unimportant things left behind.

7. *Unique element of expertise.* Employees should feel that they possess a particular expertise and know more about that unique element than anyone else.

8. *Personal accountability.* It is important to hold persons responsible for their jobs and to measure their performance objectively against predetermined standards. Personal accountability manifests itself in increasing pride in skill and service, a more constructive acceptance of errors, an increased level of creativity, and an increased sensitivity to any movement of the organization away from excellence.

When nurse-managers recognize that structuring a good and satisfying job is an important part of management, then each of these ingredients for enrichment can be transcribed into a nurse's job. A manager can furnish direct feedback by letting the nurses develop written plans based on their job descriptions and then reporting by *exception* to the manager.[8] In this way, staff nurses become the first auditors of their own performances, a situation that gives them the first opportunity to make the needed corrections.

To establish a client relationship, staff nurses should define their customers specifically by listing the key influences on why a particular patient decided to seek care at their hospital.

A learning function should be built into a job responsibility. This can be done by requiring a written plan for self-development and continued education.

As a part of job performance, nurses can prepare a schedule

of operation that shows, in the order of priority, the key milestones that can be approved and reviewed by the other team members.

Each job description should include a list of unique capabilities, areas of distinctive competence, and key skills that are needed to provide the best possible nursing care. The staff nurses can then list these unique elements of expertise as the elements relate to them personally. If any gaps exist, they can be handled as goals for personal development.

If nurses have control over their own resources, they will control the expenditures approved for carrying out their jobs in the limits of expense accounts or approved budgets. As it is, few nurses can relate the cost of equipment and supplies to the operation of the unit.

When reporting follows horizontal or diagonal lines, there is better chance for direct communication. To establish mutual goals, nurses need to deal directly with any part of the support system.

Every nurse needs to clearly understand job expectations. This requires a written description of general and specific personal accountabilities that have specific standards of measurable acceptable performance. Without standards there is no objective way to appraise performance.

In other words, a staff member will be motivated when responsibility, personal achievement, recognition, personal growth, learning, and advancement are a part of the job.

Motivation Factors

To take the guesswork out of determining if the job will provide these factors of motivation to a staff member, a research team[9] designed an instrument for comparing measures of meaningfulness of hospital jobs: the Health Professional Motivation Inventory (HPMI). Basically, it measures the potential of each job to motivate a specific group currently employed in a position. When a mismatch occurs, the scores provide clues to how the job's task assignments can be redesigned to improve motivational ability. More specifically, this is a way to look at these 12 different factors that can influence motivation:

1. Skill variety
2. Task identity
3. Task significance
4. Autonomy
5. Feedback from the job itself
6. Feedback from supervisors
7. General satisfaction
8. Supervisory satisfaction
9. Pay satisfaction
10. Individual growth need strength
11. Social need strength
12. Motivating potential

When a match occurs between the motivating potential of the job and the individual's need for achievement, the result is job satisfaction and higher levels of productivity.

Establishing job enrichment and matching growth needs with motivation potential are not done just one time; they require continuous management action. The quest to make nursing "right" should bring the job up to the level of challenge. Any nurse who has still more ability eventually will be able to demonstrate it better and win promotion to higher-level positions.

It must not be forgotton, however, that not all nurses want more responsibility, advancement, or more challenging work. Some nurses would prefer simpler jobs to jobs that are enriched. And yet, the practice of job enrichment works because it releases the motivation of a particular segment of the work force.

Releasing Motivation

Nurse-managers can be effective by mastering the concept of self-released, internal motivation. Motivation is not generated externally but comes from within the employee. Motivation cannot be imposed externally because it is an internal process. To better understand this concept, consider the motivation pyramid (Fig. 5-1). The pyramid represents a structure that relies on a layering process; each layer forms the foundation for the next. Its three-sided shape suggests the three sides of the management process: the corporation, the manager, and the staff. The pyramid demonstrates the idea that any individual release of motivation depends not only on personal needs but also on a complimentary linking with the needs of the corporation and the manager.

Maslow's Needs	**Herzberg's Motivators**	
Self-actualization	Creativity Experimentation	Meaningfulness
Recognition	Competence Achievement	Recognition Advancement
Social needs	Affiliation Acceptance	Team membership Harmony
	Herzberg's Dissatisfers:	
Security	Security Order	Rules Fringe benefits
Physical needs	Work conditions Higher wages	Leisure

Table 5-1—Comparison of Maslow's Needs and Herzberg's Motivators

Source: Maslow A: Toward a Psychology of Being. *New York, Van Nostrand Reinhold Co, 1968. Herzberg F: One more time: How do you motivate an employee?* Harvard Bus Rev, *January/February 1968; pp 58-69.*

The first or bottom layer of the pyramid is composed of the unique and individualized background of each person, the work background. The effective manager is aware (1) that each employee has unique motivating factors, (2) that no two persons are alike, and (3) that handling of life events differs with each person. In addition to the essential skills, abilities, job expectations, and professional values, careful attention must be given to successes and failures in past job experiences. Careful assessment of biographical history, abilities, and motives will help the nurse-manager create a challenging job situation and work climate that promotes self-initiating behavior and, consequently, job satisfaction.

The second layer in the motivational pyramid takes into account the preconceptions each person brings to work. Before starting a job, every employee has certain ideas about what the job will be like and what is expected for the employee's own growth and job satisfaction. Often these preconceptions do not agree with the reality the employee encounters on the job. Subsequently, situations occur that could have been remedied if the manager had defined clearly what the employee's duties included and explained why the first few months on the job may be filled with many boring assignments. When a staff member has a more accurate perception of the job, there will be less frustration and a greater chance for self-released motivation.

The third layer of the pyramid deals with the worth of the work as perceived by the individual employee. Work worth is the value of the job measured in terms of its qualities and the esteem in which it is held. When work worth is high, the release of motivation will be high because it is directly related to the amount of worth or good an employee sees in that employee's work. Work should complement an individual's concept of self and be relevant to the desire to make a significant contribution. When an employee's concept of self is expanded and complemented by the work itself, the release of motivation is increased.

The fourth layer of the pyramid deals with the feeling of

association with work. Self-released motivation exists in direct proportion to the degree of association a person feels with work. Work association depends on the three *Bs*—belonging, being, and becoming. A sense of belonging, an acceptance by the organization, is enriched when an individual feels that others in the group are aware of the importance of personal work. For staff nurses a nurse-manager's recognition is vital and meaningful, but group acceptance and recognition enhance motivational release.

The fifth and top layer of the pyramid is concerned with the need of each individual to feel important. The question is, How does a nurse-manager generate a feeling of personal importance in a job? It seems that a person's sense of importance is directly related to the influence felt through the job. It is up to the nurse-manager to establish many opportunities for a staff member to exercise influence. Directly soliciting advice and intently listening to suggestions from staff members let them know that they are an important segment in the decision-making process. The more importance felt by the staff, the more motivation is released.

Employees are motivated when their manager sees them, treats them, and communicates with them as being capable of performance excellence. Managers should treat and approach employees through the employees' self-perceptions. Assignments and the work itself become challenging and motivating when they are equal to a person's self-perceived abilities and self-worth. Assignments lose their motivational appeal when they are perceived as being below personally estimated ability, training, or experience backgrounds. When nurses see an increase in their self-respect and self-worth as a result of caring for patients and as a result of a healthy relationship with their manager, motivation is released. The challenge of today's nurse-manager is to establish a motivation-releasing climate.

One mark of a motivation-releasing climate is mutually determined goals. When this approach is combined with the nurse-manager's awareness of staff members' personal needs to participate and influence, a situation exists in which work goals are relevant to both staff and manager.

The nurse-manager should sit down regularly with staff members to develop realistic well-defined goals that call for honest contributions, not busy work. This calls for complete openness in which there are no hidden job expectations on either side.

In other words, the primary function of a nurse-manager is to ensure that the external circumstances, the style, the climate, and the opportunities of the work environment all relate positively to the needs and desires of staff members.

Now is the time to give up the notion that a manager can motivate the staff. Motivation is already in each person. Motivation is not a manipulation, nor is it caused by management. Motivation results from a close relationship between what an individual expects and needs in work and what is actually found. How well hospital nurses care for their patients depends on how well managers release the nurses' motivation.

To effectively lead and manage others, nurse-managers must gain an overall understanding of releasing motivation in an individual human being and knowledge about how to develop power strategies.

References

1. Price J: *The Study of Nursing Turnover*. Ames, Iowa, Iowa State University Press, 1977.
2. Kase S, Swenson B: Cost of hospital sponsored orientation and inservice education for registered nurses in *Health Manpower References*. US Dept of Health, Education, and Welfare, 1976, vol 77, p 25.
3. Chung H: *Motivational Theories and Practices*. Columbus, Ohio, Grid Inc, 1977.
4. Silber MB, Sherman VC: *Managerial Performance and Promotability*. Mt Prospect, Ill, Beta Group Ltd, 1983.
5. Maslow A: *Toward a Psychology of Being*. New York, Van Nostrand Reinhold Co, 1968.
6. Herzberg F: One more time: How do you motivate employees? *Harvard Bus Rev*, January/February 1968, pp 58-69.
7. Herzberg F: *The Managerial Choice—To Be Efficient and To Be Human*. Homewood, Ill, Dow Jones-Irwin, 1976.
8. Randolph RM: *Thank God It's Monday*. Englewood Cliffs, NJ, Institute for Business Planning Inc, 1982.
9. Guthrie MB, Mauer G, Zawacki RA, et al: Productivity: How much does this job mean? *Nurs Management*, February 1985, pp 16-20.

Chapter 6

Developing Power Strategies

Power-oriented people are positive. They have learned the lesson that power is the reality of life in the organization. McClelland and Burnham,[1] wrote about the two dimensions of human needs: The first is the need for dominance, or the need for power; the second is the need for love, or the need for affiliation. Persons who seem to make it more quickly to the top are power-oriented and have a relatively low need for affiliation.

Michael Korda, in his book *Power*,[2] stated that power is something that persons must give to themselves. It can never be given to them because if they accept power, they are in debt, owing something to the person who gave it to them. Power must be taken and asserted ethically.

The Meaning of Power

To many nurses, power is a four-letter word, and inconsistent with the values in nursing. However, power, achievement, and affiliation are all factors of managerial effectiveness. Contrary to what nurses might think, a good manager is not one who needs personal achievement or who is people-oriented, but one who likes power.[1]

Power people are dominant, but they are not domineering. Persons who get ahead are not afraid to risk their power. Some nurse-managers are afraid of being successful. They even divert successful outcomes when they are on the verge of success because of the risk associated with the power of the final decisions.

Power needs are dominant. Ordering of values often may spell the difference between professional effectiveness and career-performance failure. Sometimes a person will say, "If I only had more political clout around here, I could get something done for a change." In essence, this person is saying that if more power were available, achieving success would be easy. This expression of a need for power often alerts other managers to be anxious about their own power bases. It indicates a threat to their own needs for personal dominance in relationships. When this happens, the established manager becomes alienated from both the person and the purpose. This is not to say that a nurse-manager should not have power in the hospital organization, but an apparently greater emphasis on power rather than on achievement can be a self-induced handicap that interferes with upward career movement.

The effective nurse-manager examines and confronts the need for power and with finesse conveys the idea that patient-oriented achievement is at the heart of the matter. There must be no hint of domination in a relationship. Peer relationships are built through consultative guidance, not through efforts to be domineering.

Power effectiveness puts the solution to a problem into the other person's frame of reference, values, vocabulary, and operating needs. The nurse-manager must think in terms of cost as well as payoff, specifically the cost to the other person. It is an accepted fact that the medical records or laboratory manager has little or no interest in a payoff for the nurse-manager. The important point is whether the other managers perceive that the nurse-manager has a genuine concern about their needs and their career effectiveness. When the nurse-manager persuades the other managers in terms of their values, their problems, and their needs, an effective power strategy will have been learned.

Power is founded and framed on healthy self-esteem. The self-assured nurse-manager is a person who is willing to explore, redefine relationships, and assume the risk of continually looking within the self. Self-esteem generates power within a person. The powerful person is a strong person whose self-esteem rises from an awareness of personal strengths. These personal strengths are manifest in three characteristics: energy, strength, and action. These are also the behaviors necessary to affect, influence, and change human relations.

The most important and unyeilding necessity of organizational life is not human relations, better communication, or employee participation, but power—or the capacity to modify the conduct of others while avoiding the modification of one's own behavior. Power is acquired, not given, and essentially is held by shrewdness.[3]

The Rights and Responsibilities of Power

Along with power comes specific rights and responsibilities:

1. Each person has the right to judge his or her personal behavior and feelings—and the responsibility for those acts.
2. Each person has the right to choose—and the responsibility for those choices.
3. Each person has the right to say no—and the responsibility for any disagreement.
4. Each person has the right to make a request of another—as long as it is clear that the other has the right to say no.
5. Each person has the right to contradict—and the responsibility for the anger and irritation that being contradictory may cause in others.
6. Each person has the right to challenge—and the responsibility for definition and clarification.

7. Each person has the right to change his or her mind—
    and the responsibility for any difference in bargaining
    power.
8. Each person has the right to define compromise, fair-
    ness, and usefulness—and the responsibility to consider
    both sides.
9. Each person has the right to discount desires and pref-
    erences of others—and the responsibility to explain
    such decisions.
10. Each person has the right not to find solutions for
    another's problems—and the responsibility to accept
    the consequences of such action.

If these statements seem to contradict or oppose an intuitive
belief system, this situation illustrates the paradox of power.
When Randolph[4] discussed this paradox of power, he pointed out
that management must be reliable and trustworthy (ie, responsible). When power is viewed in the context of responsibility, it
implies service more than mastery. When nurse-managers
approach their jobs from this point of view, they attract a natural kind of spontaneous power, even more power than they need
to accomplish their goals. The point is that any organization
consists only of people. Therefore, mutual trust, respect, and
confidence must be derived from a belief in the fundamental
reliability of people. It is up to the nurse-manager to understand
the paradox of power and meet its inherent responsibilities.

Sources of Power

Power depends on a relationship between managers and
staff members. This relationship provides the sources of power
for the manager. Although many possible sources can be identified, French and Raven[5] distinguished five: reward power, coercive power, legitimate power, referent power, and expert power.
Chances to build on each of these sources of power occur every

day in the life of a nurse-manager. Here are a few examples:

Reward power arises from staff members' perceptions of the manager's ability to give out rewards. For example, top management has observed that one nurse-manager frequently was honored at luncheons and his crew were always willing to work overtime without complaints. After a little investigation, it was discovered that he recognized and praised his staff members for any of their contributions. In one incident he not only wrote a personal note of thanks for his ward clerk's suggestion (about purchasing supplies at a lower cost) but also published that letter in the hospital newsletter. Needless to say, staff members responded to this nurse-manager's rewards, and he developed a base of referent power.

Coercive power comes from staff members' perceptions that the manager has the ability to punish. Even though a nurse-manager does not like to think that a power base is built on the act of punishment, there comes a time when a staff member must be fired. After careful documentation of the problems that had arisen from clashing interpersonal relationships, a nurse-manager confronted a staff nurse with the evidence and offered the choice of resignation or termination. The issue here is not the firing but the reaction from other staff members. When they realized that the nurse in question was no longer a team member, they agreed with the action, which gave more credit and respect to the nurse-manager. This is an example of how the ability to punish with congruent perceptions raised the power base.

Legitimate power stems from staff members' perceptions that the manager has a legitimate right to prescribe behavior. Whether it is a pattern for staffing or requests for doing things a certain way, a manager has the legal right to do these things. When the CEO asks that all nurse-managers keep project lists and identify performance goals, they do it (even though they might perceive such activities as busy work). In other words, they do it because the top management said so. That is legitimate power.

Referent power is generated from staff members' identification with the manager. When a nurse-manager gave staff members the opportunity to write operational goals and develop a mission statement, they responded by not only developing their own goals but also designing specific goals for their nurse-manager. They suggested that she increase patient volume, increase contributions, and develop a name identity in the community while they would take care of the patients by shortening the patients' waiting time, clarifying communication with physicians, and responding to patients' specific needs. This shows how a nurse-manager can increase referent power by giving staff members the opportunity for autonomy. They liked what she had done.

Expert power is derived from the staff members' perceptions that the manager has some special knowledge. Even though a manager may be perceived as a likable person, the "boss," a "rewarder," or a "punisher," the need to demonstrate personal ability still exists. A newly employed nurse-manager in a nursing home discovered that the cardiac monitor and the defibrillator were not being used. Even though the technology was available, staff members seemed to avoid using the equipment. The nurse-manager then introduced lessons on basic arrhythmias at each staff meeting. As staff members became involved in learning more about heart physiology and what could be seen on a monitor, they recognized that their nurse-manager was knowledgeable about cardiac care. In this way, by demonstrating her expertise, the nurse-manager added to her power base.

Each of these power sources can be enhanced by using three informal strategies. Every manager needs visibility, sponsorship, and a distinctive style. To attain visibility, the nurse-manager does a lot of visiting to collect political data, acquires responsibility, selects the work arenas that can be seen, and offers to be the messenger for information.

Sponsorship is cultivating persons who are at the top. To show loyalty, which is the link between power persons, a manager must know the value structure of the sponsor. A secured power base comes to the manager who walks in the power shadows of at least two persons.

The third way of enhancing a power base is to develop a distinguishing style of management. The nurse-manager who has a flare for matching staff members with the jobs to be done or the goals to be accomplished will increase power. Staff members who get to do what they want to do often perceive this situation as a reward. When the nurse-manager delegates some of the responsibility of management to the staff, expert power is increased because staff members perceive the manager as having a special ability in dealing with people. The nurse-manager also will avoid becoming isolated from employees because losing the personal touch will produce suspicion and loss of legitimate power. These strategies for power work well when specific skills and tactics are developed.

Development of Power Skills

Del Bueno[6] suggested that developing power skills can lead to success. If her ideas are put into the context of hospital management, the following examples indicate some specific strategies nurse-managers can use to develop power:

- *Build a personal team.* When a nurse-manager accepts a new position, there is a risk because those employees inherited from another manager may be unhappy enough to engage in sabotage. One step a new nurse-manager must take is to know each team member. It is necessary to define why members are satisfied and why they are unhappy with their positions. If any of them suggests that long job tenure should have been rewarded by a managerial position, then that person must be recognized as a potential threat. Recognizing the reason for discontent and then delegating some managerial responsibility to that person will ease the tension and enlist that person as a team player.

- *Choose the second in command carefully*. A number two person who is aggressive and expressing a need for power to accomplish assigned tasks is probably expressing a need to dominate. This does not encourage team building. Teams are built with those people who subordinate personal feats and glory for the good of the team.
- *Establish alliances with both superiors and peers*. The nurse-manager must take plenty of time to determine the expectations and motives of both staff members and superiors. Then it is up to the manager to establish friendships with those who have a similar value system and wish to accomplish the hospital goals in a similar fashion.
- *Use all possible channels of communication*. Every nurse-manager needs to use both upward and downward communication. The grapevine and spies supply a lot of information. It is up to the nurse-manager to listen to the concerns of employees at all levels. Often subordinates do not have the chance to interact directly, so they depend on intermediaries to convey their concerns. More specifically, it is often the secretary or the ward clerk who hears about problems and relays these concerns to the nurse-manager.
- *Know when to be fair to subordinates*. Fairness does not mean delegating authority to the unhappy manipulators who want to take over management. Sometimes not all requests can be granted. Being fair may mean setting limits rather than delegating authority. As an example, when a group of coronary care nurses were given the autonomy to develop a cardiac rehabilitation program within the confines of a given budget, they were not permitted to hire a dietitian. Their request would have exceeded the budget and encroached on the job of the nurse-manager.
- *Be aware of the pervasive influence of powerful people*. Being aware of the biases of persons in high places,

nurse-managers cannot be naive about how decisions are made. They must recognize that even whims of the powerful can be granted.

- *Know what takes priority.* The goal-oriented nurse-manager can determine what tasks or services take precedence.
- *Be courteous.* Every nurse-manager must recognize that courtesy builds referent power. When others do not feel respect and consideration, there is always a chance for retaliation.
- *Maintain a flexible position.* By now, every nurse-manager should know that this strategy makes compromise possible along with skillful adaptation to changing circumstances.
- *Use deception judiciously.* Another power skill to be developed is knowing that sometimes it is unwise to divulge personal preferences over organizational goals. At other times it is unwise to let others know favorite personal power strategies. These things are simply kept to oneself.
- *Use passive resistance when under pressure from demands that cannot be challenged openly.* Nurse-managers soon learn that a delay in the action may be the only way to protect their best interests. Sometimes no action is the best action.
- *Project an image of status, power, and material success.* Nurse-managers are measured by the way they live, act, and dress. A modest, shy individual might be mistaken for a person without any power or influence. Others relate to a person according to the way that person dresses, speaks on the telephone, phrases a letter, and greets others. To be a success, a person must act and look like success.

Developing these skills and tactics will make the nurse-manager a power-projecting person.

Power-Projecting Persons

Certain behaviors are expected of power-projecting nurse-managers:

- They are not frightened by closeness, confrontation, choice, or change.
- They can spell out acceptable compromises each step of the way.
- They can assume a steady posture and a quiet stare, hesitate, and be silent at the risk of being disliked.
- They do not take it personally when they are called immobile, impassive, impatient, or indifferent.
- They can say no without an explanation, or they can give no answer.
- They never ignore a put-down and set limits early on any troublemaker.
- Above all, when they are dealing with conflict, they concentrate on the issue, not the emotion.

These personality characteristics distinguish effective nurse-managers' dispositions and mark them as valuable to the organization.

Personal power skills also can help make a person more effective. Diane Kellogg, assistant professor of management at Bentley College, has categorized personal power skills into likability, connections, reciprocity, expert power, and the ability to reward.[7] When these skills are combined with top job performance, a difference can be made in a manager's career.

Likability is composed of style, confidence, ability to persuade, and integrity. Style can be defined as the way a nurse-manager deals with co-workers, the ability to fit in or the ability to make co-workers feel at ease with the manager's approach. Nurse-managers erase "my demands" and "my expectations" from their vocabulary.[8]

The power of persuasion and confidence are important aspects of likability, but without integrity, a warm, open style can be interpreted as manipulation. On the other hand, sometimes the ability to project confidence is interpreted as aggressiveness. Unfortunately, a double standard still exists on the amount of aggressiveness that can be used by men and by women. In some organizations, men are allowed more aggressiveness than women are. In other words, a man can still be likable if he is aggressive, but a woman must handle aggressiveness with velvet gloves.

Likability creates mixed feelings in some women because they want their successes attributed to their abilities, not their personalities. This is erroneous because the heart of management is person-to-person transactions.

In other women likability causes unrest because these women fear that their personal warmth may be misinterpreted as sexual gestures. These are legitimate fears, but more problems are generated when a manager is not relaxed or amusing.

Connections are important because making and maintaining contact with colleagues, inside and outside the hospital, cannot be left to chance. Connections make it possible to gain information about the achievers of the organization and about new ideas and new proposals.

The best connections make giving and collecting favors a possibility. Reciprocity, however, must be dealt with in a subtle way by making it clear that the manager possesses something of value, that it is worth sharing, and that the other person needs to take the time to listen. Developing trade-offs is a shrewd power tactic because if nurse-managers cannot develop innovations on their own, they can trade for the support they need from co-workers.

Expertise beyond the prerequisites of a job can increase personal power. Specialized knowledge can be planned or unplanned. The point is, a nurse-manager's personal influence is increased when others come to the manager for advice.

Rewards also will increase a manager's personal influence. Raises and promotions are not the only ways to reward staff members. Praise, information, introductions, attention, assignments, and assistance will make a person feel good and be willing to work hard for the giver. Adept reward givers always find capable persons to work with them and accomplish the company's goals.

Likability, connections, reciprocity, expertise, and reward combined with attitude, luck, tactics, and personality combined with excellent job performance can bring success only when combined with habits of power.

Habits of Power

To paraphrase Harragan,[8] somewhere in line with job performance, nurse-managers must develop the habits of power if they hope to advance into positions of real responsibility. Exerting power and authority easily and naturally is a new experience for most nurses. Like any other skill it must be learned and practiced.

A promotion to supervise and manage an operation brings physical and psychologic exposure, but this is the time to demonstrate future potential by using influence and exerting power. The new subordinates and the new superiors will be watching to judge every action. Too often nurses entering management jobs fail to perceive that their priorities have changed and plunge headlong into the task itself, trying desperately to prove their worthiness and demonstrate their abilities, not recognizing that their task has changed—from doing the work to getting others to do the work for them.

Intent on proving themselves to superiors and accustomed to being in a subordinate position, new nurse-managers may lose sight of the goals of the organization. In other words, the immediate concern for the manager is the action going on with the staff. It is up to the manager to recognize the power base, delegate authority, direct the tasks, and then see how well the staff functions. As Kanter[9] so aptly put it, what it takes to get the organization up and running is essentially the same two things all vehicles need: a person in the driver's seat and a source of power.

Delegating authority and sharing responsibility is really sharing power. In this situation staff members are encouraged to disagree and get into problem solving with the manager rather than carry out orders obediently. However, some nurse-managers are reluctant to do this because they feel that they do not have power commensurate with their responsibilities. Such reluctance, according to Bradford and Cohen,[10] makes sense only if the manager assumes (1) that the amount of power is fixed (so that by sharing some with staff members, the manager ends up with less) and (2) that staff members will use their increased influence to block attainment of department goals. From one point of view, both assumptions are valid. If the nurse-manager and the staff are in a dispute that only one of them can win, increasing the staff's power may be to the manager's disadvantage. On the other hand, if power is defined as the ability to get things done, then there can be enabling power as well as restrictive power. A nurse-manager uses power and influence by increasing staff members' work responsibilities and assisting them to be more competent.

According to Bradford's and Cohen's principles,[10] it is up to the nurse-manager to understand the two faces worn by power and influence. If the emphasis is on restrictive power—on increasing the discrepancy between the manager's level of influence and the staff's—the final effect may be to decrease the amount of the manager's influence. On the other hand, if the manager places primary importance on enabling power and seeks to increase the ability of staff members to be influential, the final effect can be to increase the manager's power.

The explanation for this apparent contradiction is that most healthy adults seek to avoid being dependent. They are willing to be under the power and influence of another, but only when they can retain some sense of autonomy. When power is increased beyond interdependence to dependence, there will be resistance, which may take the form of constant disagreement. When persons feel that they have some control over what will happen to them, they are more open to influence.

When a nurse-manager increases the influence of staff members, they are more likely to consider the manager's ideas rather than resist them. When the staff's responsibility is increased, commitment is increased also.

In summary, manager power can increase in three specific ways:

1. When there is a sense of obligation felt by staff members for the effort the nurse-manager makes in staff development
2. When staff resistance is decreased by making assignments according to the staff members' needs
3. When the manager is on the staff's side

Power is not a fixed entity. In many hospitals, there is too little power. Nurse-managers who sense they are in low power situations will be hesitant about giving staff members increased influence in the decision-making process. Yet the more power that is given away, the stronger the manager's power base becomes. Staff members who feel themselves a part of the influencing process are more committed to the hospital's goals. On the other hand, staff members with feelings of low power will resist the power of others. The best way for a nurse-manager to have a solid power base is to increase staff responsibility and influence.

References

1. McClelland DC, Burnham DH: Power is the great motivator. *Harvard Bus Rev*, March/April 1976, pp 100-110.
2. Korda M: *Power*. New York, Ballantine Books Inc, 1981.
3. McMurrary RN: Power and the ambitious executive. *Harvard Bus Rev*, November/December 1973, pp 140-145.
4. Randolph RM: *Thank God It's Monday*. Englewood Cliffs, NJ, Institute for Business Planning Inc, 1982.
5. French JRP Jr, Raven B: The bases of power, in Cartwright D (ed): *Studies in Social Power*. Ann Arbor, Mich, Institute for Social Research, 1959, pp 150-165.
6. Del Bueno DJ: Power and politics in organizations. *Outlook*, May/June 1986, pp 124-128.
7. Burns C: The extra edge. *Savvy*, December 1982, pp 38-43.
8. Harragan BL: *Games Mother Never Taught You*. New York, Warner Books Inc, 1977.
9. Kanter RM: *The Change Masters*. New York, Simon & Schuster Inc, 1983.
10. Bradford DL, Cohen AR: *Managing for Excellence*. New York, John Wiley & Sons Inc, 1984.

Chapter 7

The Nurse-Manager as Change Agent

Change is an inevitable, complex, and continuous process that affects everybody. For many managers difficulty with change stems from an incomplete knowledge of the inherent properties that characterize change. Change is a function of time. Nothing remains static. Everything that is occurring within and around humans exists in a state of flux. Change is unavoidable, and it affects everyone. Change must be recognized, talked about, and accepted by both nurse-managers and staff members. Persons are involved in change whether they like it or not. It is a process present in every facet of life. Change provides difficulties in its own right for the individual or group of individuals involved.

The Nature of Change

Being aware that persons experience difficulties with change and try to resist it adds insight into why bringing about change is difficult. An important factor in producing resistance is the psychologic one, which can be seen as encompassing the personal needs, fears, and attitudes of an individual. When persons join a health system, they do so because they expect to satisfy some of their personal needs. One is providing an income for themselves and their families. Other important needs include the need for security and the need to give meaning to their job life. These needs can be considered basic, and tampering with their source is viewed as posing a threat to the security of the individual involved.

The threat to self-vested needs produced when a nursing division attempts to incorporate change turns into fear. This fear can originate from management's failure to clearly and adequately communicate what changes are being made and what effects these changes will have on which employees. Insufficient communication gives rise to self-concern and fear of loss. Employees begin asking themselves, "Can I do the job?" Persons fear the unknown because of the lack of predictability and the perceived inability to control their own destinies. Unpredictability and ambiguity spawn adverse attitudes.

Attitudes are a relatively enduring disposition to behave or react in a certain way. The behavior chosen by a person to reflect attitudes toward change depends on that person's disposition to change and on an evaluation of the immediate consequences (what may be lost by resisting the impending change). A nurse's attitude towards change is affected by the trust in management and by the work group within the hospital in which the nurse is a member. Work groups influence a person's attitude toward change by exerting social pressure; persons listen to others in the group because being part of a group assures security, power, and self-esteem.

Acting in conjunction with the threat to self-esteem is the job itself, which is composed of the various factors that go into making up the actual tasks and the work environment in which it exists. Change may be a threat to the earnings received or to the status, power, and recognition of the job. Other factors threatened by change are the chance for professional advancement, the removal of familiar and favorable working conditions, and the loss of membership in a particular group. In other words, there can be a threat to a nurse's self-esteem because of changes in nursing itself, and there can be threats to a nurse's salary and status as a team leader. Attempts to change these job factors without adequate justification can lead to resistance and negative reactions on the part of the employee. An insensitive nurse-manager fails to realize that employees acquire a vested interest in their work and that any change in it becomes personal. Nurses think of their jobs and their work environment as their life space and as belonging to them, not to the hospital.

Change is not neutral in the eyes of nurses because it is interpreted personally by them. A manager's sensitivity can mean the difference between success or failure of change acceptance. If a nurse-manager hopes to avoid many difficulties, attempts should be made to view the impact of change from the perspective of the nurses who are to be involved. After all, they are the ones who will determine the degree of success of the impending change.

The extent to which nurse-managers consider the perspectives of their staff members when introducing change is a reflection of the management climate of the hospital. Attitude climates differ widely among hospitals and produce different sensitivities toward the incorporation of change. Some nurse-managers exhibit participative styles; others exhibit nonparticipative styles. These styles can be thought of as the personality of the organization.

When instituting change, participative nurse-managers invest the time to explain not only what the change is but also why a specific change is needed. For employees to accept and support a change they must have an emotional reason to institute it. Progress-and-growth concepts are too general and help very little when a manager is trying to justify a specific change that affects only certain nursing units or specific employees. To gain emotional support for a proposed change from those involved, the purpose, impact, and intent of the change must be disclosed and discussed as relevant and necessary for each person involved. Explanation and justification are powerful and important management tools.

The nurse-manager who institutes change unannounced, unexplained, and unjustified will be viewed with suspicion by the employees. Under these circumstances change becomes a threat, and persons will go to great lengths to block or stall it.

The announcement of change should be simple, direct, and honest. The information should be factual and sufficiently detailed to minimize undue apprehension and distortion of the situation. At the same time, it should provide knowledge of the purposes and the steps to be used to achieve the objectives. Whether all information about the change should be furnished at one time or little by little at different times (the timing of the announcement) depends mainly on the specific situation.

The initial announcement should be used as a vehicle to solicit suggestions. When persons are directly involved in the process, change becomes more meaningful because they experience personal identification with the organization's goal. Their commitment to immediate change is strengthened, and their commitment to their future is assured. Participation reduces resistance.

Employees are less resistant when they are kept informed about what is taking place and encouraged to take part in it. Remember, work provides a dual purpose; it provides a means for support and, at the same time, gives a personal sense of meaning. Any threat to work endangers the worker's total existence. It is no wonder that employees actively resist any effort to change their work environment.

Encouraging and accepting employees' participation in changes in their work need not be a threat to management. Nurse-managers should not fear allowing staff members to aid in change. Instead, the managers should use their personnel resources as wisely as they use their physical or financial resources. Establishing a two-way flow of information and ideas with the staff members increases the identification each person has with the needed changes. Staff members want to feel that their suggestions are being recognized and used. Adding meaning to a person's job life by enhancing that person's importance mutually benefits everyone involved.

Listening to those who are directly involved and affected by the change can stimulate insight and information that stems from day-in and day-out experiences that no one else has. For the most part, many staff nurses are well aware of where changes are needed long before management is. Too many nurse-managers, however, have the idea that it is "bad business" to ask their staff members for information about a better, easier, and more efficient method to perform a task. This leads to inefficient methods and reduces performance and increases cost. Nurse-managers must recognize that they are like their nursing personnel because both have similar personal needs. Each group needs to feel mutually compatible. One easy way to bring about compatible change is through open communication.

Nurse-managers should promote the flow of ideas, needs, and feelings between themselves and staff members. Doing this on a day-to-day basis facilitates change. Keeping in touch or staying in tune through gradual changes and their evolution is the most significant means to remain viable.

Planning Change

Many social processes exist within the hospital: the interactions between individuals and between groups, the way information is transmitted, the unwritten ground rules, the attitudes of persons, and the way work is done. When change is introduced, any one or several of these processes can be affected. Change does not come easily because, in reality, it is a minor revolution. When change is not planned, it can erupt into a civil war. Beckard[1] suggested a sequence of steps for the process of planning change (Exhibit 7-1). Most of these steps are developed by asking questions.

Step 1: Define the change problem.
Step 2: Identify the change process.
Step 3: Determine readiness.
Step 4: Determine capability.
Step 5: Identify resources.
Step 6: Determine intermediate strategies.
Step 7: State the plan of action.
Step 8: Determine the target.
Step 9: Take action.
Step 10: Maintain change via continued feedback.

Exhibit 7-1—Steps in the Process of Planning Change

Source: Beckard R: Strategies for large system change. Sloan Management Rev, *Winter 1975, pp 43-55.*

Step 1 is to define the change problem by asking these questions:

- Is it a morale problem?
- Is it the way work is done?
- Is it the communication system?
- Is it the reporting system?
- Is it the structure or location of the decision making?
- Is it the effectiveness of the top team?
- Is it interlevel relationships?
- Is it the way goals are set?
- Is it something else?

These questions consider many parts of the organization in an effort to uncover problem areas.

Step 2 is to identify the change process. This can be done by asking if the primary initial change requires a difference of

- Attitudes? If so, whose?
- Behavior? By whom and to what?
- Knowledge and understanding? If so, where?
- Organizational procedures? If so, where?
- Practices and ways to work?

After each of these questions has been answered, the next item to be determined is the rank ordering of the various types of change needed. Which should be changed first?

On the basis of the priority established by ranking, each type of change requires a different approach and a different plan. For instance, if knowledge needs to be changed, then an educational process must be designed. If procedures need changing, then a restructuring of the type of organization might be designed. A perceived need for change in attitudes or behavior might indicate a concentrated effort toward creating a different type of climate.

Step 3 is to determine the readiness for change. Persons should be asked directly the following:

- Are you satisfied with the way things are being done around here?
- If you are not satisfied, do you have an idea about what could be changed?
- Do you have an idea where we should start?
- If you are not satisfied, are you ready to work hard to bring things to your satisfaction?

These questions try to determine the readiness of staff members, the attitudinal or motivational energy available to bring about the prescribed change. Change will not occur without enough dissatisfaction, an idea of what "would be" if change were successful, an awareness of starting points, and an idea of the amount of energy that it will take to make the change. If the nurse-manager does not discover a readiness for change, three actions can be taken.

First, if most of the staff members really are not dissatisfied with the present state of things, then the action is to increase their level of dissatisfaction. Second, if there is plenty of dissatisfaction but no clear picture of the desired state, then a person of authority should define the desired state. Third, if dissatisfaction and a clear picture of a desired state exist, but practical first steps are missing, then an experimental unit could begin the change activities.

Step 4 is to determine the capability for change. Capability is defined as the physical, financial, or organizational means to make the change. Questions to be asked include the following:

- Are there funds?
- Is management willing to allocate resources?
- Does each designated leader have the personal capabilities for change?

Answers to these questions will determine if change is feasible.

Step 5 is to identify resources and motivations for the change. Nurse-managers should ask themselves

- Am I in agreement with the prescribed changes?
- Who will be my support group?
- Am I personally dissatisfied enough to exert energy beyond the usual expected performance?

Without personal involvement by the manager no change plan can even be designed let alone instigated.

Step 6 is to determine the intermediate strategy. Questions for this step include the following:

- What is the readiness of each group to be influenced?
- What is the accessibility of each unit?
- What is the linkage of each unit to the hospital?

Even before the change process is started, the nurse-manager finds out the best way to get the unit ready, determines those persons who are easy to get along with, and decides on a method of linking their efforts to the proposed change.

Step 7 is to state the plan of action. After the organization, managers, staff, and work have been studied, here are some possible actions:

- Is the plan changing the climate of the organization?
- Is the plan changing managerial style?
- Is the plan changing the organizational structure to relate to the way work is actually done?
- Is the plan changing the ways the work is done to improve meaningfulness and efficiency?
- Is the plan changing the reward system so that it is consistent with the work?

It takes careful deliberation to determine the action. The interrelatedness of systems and subsystems within the hospital means that any change anywhere will cause a ripple effect.

Step 8 is to determine the target. Here are some possible choices:

- The top team
- A pilot project
- Ready units (those whose staff members and managers are ready for change)
- Hurting units (those with environmental discomforts)
- The reward system

Hitting the right target improves the chances of implementing change successfully.

Step 9 is to take action. Once the need for change has been identified, readiness has been determined, personal and organizational resources have been identified, the type of action has been selected, and the target has been determined, the plan for change is presented very carefully to staff.

The last step, step 10, is to maintain change by means of continued feedback. Keeping staff members informed about the progress of change is as important as determining the readiness for change. This can be accomplished by periodic team meetings and discussion sessions with interdependent units.

To clarify this process of planning change, consider the problem that hospitals have with Medicare payments based on DRGs. Hospitals suddenly found that their revenues would be decreased to a national norm. This change in reduced dollars led to the development of a system to reduce costs and maximize resources. In defining the change problem, it was decided that the most efficient way to provide reduced costs was to decrease the number of days a patient stayed in the hospital.

This change process has required a difference in attitudes on the part of the nurses as to how to decrease costs and what constitutes necessary care, as well as an understanding of the reason for shorter hospital stays.

In most cases, nurses simply are not ready to expend the amount of energy needed for change. Dissatisfaction is ample, but there is no clear picture of why the "new way" is necessary. This is where the nurse-manager spends a lot of time in gentle persuasion and in defining exactly what cost-effective quality care means.

In determining capability for change, nurse-managers usually find that funds and resources are available but that personal knowledge of change theory is lacking. However, when the nurse-manager's own resources and motivations for change are identified, and the amount of congruency found between the values of the manager and health care system is great, there is a strong indication that the nurse-manager will be an advocate for change. (It is possible to be a successful change agent without a formal theory background.)

In the problem under consideration the next step is determining readiness. If the staff remains dissatisfied, and yes, even disgruntled, without motivation after an explanation of the relationship between short stays and cost-effective care, then it is time to find one unit in which improvement activities can begin.

The specific plan of action is to change the way patients are cared for, so there is a special effort to improve the meaningfulness and the efficiency of the work. The target for this plan is a unit that is ready. Once the plan for change has started, it is up to the nurse-manager to keep all the units informed about the progress and success in managing to provide an excellent quality of care even when hospital stays are shortened.

Presenting the Proposal

The number of obstacles and the length of time between change and its eventual implementation may dampen initial enthusiasm for seeing the change through. With some thought and planning, obstacles to proposals for change can be overcome. It is possible to convince top management and staff personnel that change is worth making.

The first point nurse-managers must remember about getting a change idea accepted is that they should not try to bulldoze it through. Instead they should try to anticipate higher management's needs and preferences. The strategy is look for ways to accommodate any tender spots without materially affecting the worth of the proposal. Instead of marching around in full battle armor, managers should be receptive to suggestions on ways to modify the proposed change. They should use ingenuity to figure out ways to modify it so that even if one of its elements is rejected, the others will be accepted. When trying to get a change idea accepted, the adage to remember is that half a loaf is better than none. Getting half of the change proposal accepted puts the nurse-manager in a win-win situation rather than a win-lose struggle in which everything could be lost.

The second point to remember is that change ideas should be offered in the form of a proposal. Any ideas about change should be presented to top management in an interesting, clear, and understandable way. Here are some suggestions for writing a convincing proposal.

- *Simplify the written proposal to the point at which it can be understood.* A proposal filled with technical jargon— even when it will be read by experts—will strike a sour note with the reader. Speak first to feelings. If an appeal to expertise is necessary, it can come on a later page.
- *Put a summary and recommendations for action on page 1 of the proposal.* Do not make the reader wade through the whole package to find out what the proposal is.
- *Offer a number of alternative solutions.* Do not give just one suggestion on how to solve a problem. Give several— together with their possible negative or positive consequences. Presenting several approaches to a problem conveys the message that a lot of thought has been given to the problem and that there is no intent to railroad through the first idea that came along.

- *Show how the proposal can be put into effect*. It is easier to identify and describe a problem than to spell out how it should be solved. If a clear, step-by-step map of the change idea is provided, the chances for putting the proposal across are greatly enhanced.
- *Mold the presentation to fit the existing framework, terminology, and objectives of the organization*. Make sure that the proposal will mesh with existing physical conditions, work procedures, and personalities of employees who will be affected.
- *Present the proposal in such a way that top management has only to answer yes or no to it*. Careful preparation includes anticipating most of top management's questions and answering them in the document itself. All that remains is to make a decision.

Nurse-managers who use the following suggestions will enhance the chance that the change idea will be considered.

- *Get mutual identification and definition of the problem*. Meet with top management to define the causes, dimensions, and ramifications of the problem that the change idea will solve. Be sure that the problem is one of mutual concern. Do not waste time and energy on a problem that top management does not recognize.
- *Involve superiors in developing possible solutions*. Of course, top management may not have suggestions, but any suggestion is worth entertaining because participation gives top management a personal share in the undertaking.
- *Focus on the strength of the idea*. Ethically, the negative aspects of the proposal must be identified, but the strength of the idea must remain the focus.
- *Present ideas at the opportune moment*. Anticipate the time when superiors will be most receptive. Everyone has mood swings. Find out what the emotional state is before

presenting the proposal. During the development phase, alert superiors to some of the pertinent ideas. This provides an opportunity for planting seeds that will prepare the way for acceptance of the proposal.

- *Stress that an opportunity is presenting itself.* Show genuine concern about the problem. Any appeal to fear will hamper efforts to influence others. The effective change agent never strikes a note of panic and desperation, but rather one of optimism about the mutual gains to be made.

Overcoming Resistance

In the course of trying to get an idea accepted, patience often is tested. Obstacles must be dealt with, but if change is to be brought about, persistence is required. The change agent has a good reason to persist. Frequently, change is needed, but unfortunately change breeds resistance. Creating something new may mean tearing down something old. Most people fear this tearing down, and because of this fear, they fight change. The patient change agent does not give up or quit in anger or disgust. The only time to quit is when every avenue available has been tried and there is no way for recommended change to be understood. Change takes patience and perseverance.

Even though perseverance has gotten a proposal accepted, this is only half the battle. The other half is getting staff members or the persons affected by the change to accept it. No matter what the change is, persons may perceive it as dangerous or as criticism of their competence. A change in a clinical procedure, for example, might make staff members anxious about their previous abilities or performances.

Frequently, staff persons resist change because they do not want to think of themselves as cogs in a machine or creatures of someone else's whim. Resistance will intensify if they feel that they must comply simply because that is what is expected of them. In this case, they will see themselves as serfs in bondage to a feudal master, a condition that is hardly conducive to cooperation.

Resistance to change can be increased by group pressure. If a member of a team knows that others in the group oppose change, hesitation is likely, and there could be group rejection if the change idea is accepted.

Another reason for resistance to change may be the personal investment of a person's time and effort in an existing method. When it has taken months to master the particular system or clinical process slated for change, even a broadly beneficial change may seem destructive.

When change is perceived as a criticism, more compliance, a threat to group process, or a loss of invested time, there will be resistance that the nurse-manager must overcome.

To turn resistance into willing cooperation, feelings and perceptions about the change must be taken into account. Instead of pushing the change through over staff members' objections, the nurse-manager should make an appeal to their self-interests. As much as persons may like to think of themselves as rational beings, their emotions are usually the major determinants of what they do or resist doing.

The nurse-manager can help overcome resistance by taking time to find out how staff members see the proposed change, by listening to their doubts and fears. One way to get them to accept the new way is to enlist their cooperation. Here are some suggestions that nurse-managers can use to elicit the cooperation of staff members:

- *Get the group leader on the manager's side.* A first step in overcoming resistance to change is to identify the informal group leader. This is the person who can make or break planned change because the group looks to this individual for approval, advice, and protection. In fact, employees sometimes go to the group leader rather than to their supervisor with their problems. Gaining the confidence of the group leader is absolutely necessary. Planned change depends on finding out feelings, reactions, and opinions about the planned change. The group leader is the one who will influence the group's reaction to the change.

- *Communicate clearly the reasons for the change.* Address any false notions or rumors that have been built up about the anticipated change. Stress the task-centered aspect of the change so that employees will not take it personally. Try to eliminate any perceived threat, and let staff members know that their competence is respected. Involve staff members by asking for suggestions and opinions.

- *Give staff members a sense of belonging and sharing in the success of change.* The more members of a group feel that they are needed to institute the change, the more favorable they will be to the change. When they are asked about problems related to the planned change and ways to solve those problems, they will be actively participating in the change plan and may even generate some better, alternative solutions.

- *Be honest.* Openly discuss the potential pitfalls as well as the advantages involved in the change. Discuss the negative aspects to reduce the impact of staff members' objections.

- *Point out the positive side.* Emphasize achievement opportunities, possibilities for job diversification, and rewards for accomplishment. Change must be explained in terms of the staff members' goals and values. Success in persuasion will depend on the ability to discuss change in terms of the vested self-interest of the group. When self-interest is ignored, the real questions will not be answered.

- *When a change is going to be made, announce it promptly.* The worst enemy of planned change is rumor. Rumors start when management waits too long to give out crucial information about change. A blunt announcement should be avoided. It is better to discuss the problems that make the change necessary. Then, make sure that all concerned will have time to learn new methods. Employees become less afraid of change when they know that they will have time to absorb and learn.

- *Implement change in progressive stages*. When change is implemented over time, it becomes more palatable and easier to assimilate. Not only the overall plan of change should be presented but also when the changes will stop.

By now every nurse-manager is aware that sophisticated strategies for change must be planned and tactfully executed. To be effective agents for change, nurse-managers must thoroughly understand their staff. As managers establish rapport, they will explore attitudes and beliefs for potential incompatibilities with change. The first clue of discord alerts the manager to a potential staff problem. Tips on counseling the problem employee are found in the next chapter.

Reference

1. Beckard R: Strategies for large system change. *Sloan Management Rev*, Winter 1975, pp 43-55.

Chapter 8

Counseling the Problem Employee[*]

In terms of personnel costs, counseling and returning the problem employee to productivity offer the hospital and the individual the opportunity to optimize their contributions to each other and reconcile the problem within the working unit.

In the competitive, professional, intensive environment of the health care system, acquisition, development, and conservation of human resources are of paramount importance. The savings from retaining an employee rather than hiring a new one results in both money and "mental" advantages. Nonproductive time associated with job orientation and turnover costs are saved when staff problems are managed skillfully.

Recognizing the Problem Employee

Persons are regarded as problem employees for many reasons: They show a disagreeable attitude, attack authority, waste time, damage clinical supplies persistently, create friction on the work unit, antagonize others, have poor attendance records, or simply do not do their jobs. Although some employees seem to exhibit some of these behaviors some of the time, it is the degree and frequency of these disruptive actions that determine the problem employee. The question to be asked is, Do the problem behaviors occur frequently enough or endure long enough to interfere seriously with productivity or acceptance in the work group?

[*]Note: This chapter is an edited version of a previously unpublished lecture by MBS.

Solutions to employee problems are oriented toward conservation and revitalization of human assets by means of counseling, retraining, transfers, and termination (if the decision is made that the employee will not be a contributing member).

Many employee problems surface in the work experience. Human resources can be wasted by poor definition of the role nurse-managers expect an employee to play or through lack of education and practice. It can even be caused by an inadequate socialization process on the nursing unit and by interpersonal conflicts.

The nurse-manager must quickly recognize the conflict or note the potential problem employee early in the work process. Indicators are poor performance, evasiveness, defensive behavior, and poor interpersonal relationships with other members of the work unit. Promptly addressing these realities increases the probability of success in the conservation of human resources. When recruitment took place, the nurse-manager was confident the employee could do the job, so it is up to the nurse-manager to find out what went wrong.

Counseling

Nurse-managers can learn to recognize symptoms leading to problem behavior, be taught to conduct counseling interviews, and learn to know when to refer employees to a professional clinician.

Nursing units cause many tensions in the individual employee. Persons who are frustrated in their ambitions may fear they will be caught up in a hospital system so large that it does not permit them to maintain personal identity. Situations outside the job also can lead to excessive pressure and can result in problem behaviors on the job. When employees go to work, their personal problems go with them. These may be financial, family, health, or marital problems. If life pressures such as competing obligations and competition for time are great tensions for a person, that person may become a problem employee.

Jobs make both intellectual and emotional and interactional demands on an employee. Individuals bring more to a job than merely abilities, aptitudes, and experiences. They also seek satisfaction of various social, personal, and emotional needs.

Nurse-managers soon realize the visible problem of a problem employee and may try to solve it through counseling. When it comes to this point, the question of who will counsel the employee must be answered. It is a key principle in management to give the person who has immediate supervision of the problem employee the responsibility of counseling.

Nurse-managers use three approaches: direct action, reassurance, and nondirective counseling. In direct action the nurse-manager is the decision-maker for the employee and sees that each direction is carried out. If an employee has a problem, the nurse-manager gives advice. If the nurse-manager has a problem with the staff, solutions are given through direct advice. This approach assumes that advice is effective and that it will help the affected individual solve the problem. Persons rarely change their attitudes or behaviors with this kind of counseling.

To provide reassurance, the nurse-manager must find a logic to show that everything will be all right. However, many times the problem employee does not feel reassured because the employee may be agreeing with the nurse-manager only for the sake of politeness. Overwhelming reassurance from others tends to prevent a person from talking freely about the way the person really feels or from expressing personal doubts and fears.

The objective of nondirective counseling is to determine the problem. Once emotions are reduced, problem employees are able to get away from their own protective feelings and look for the source of change. As long as it is expected or believed that someone else must change, they will not address and solve the problems. The responsibility for dealing with what needs to be changed must be accepted by the individual who has the problem. The nurse-manager can help the frustrated staff member locate the problem by assisting in an exploration of the real or imaginary changes. The manager guides the individual to find alternative solutions that are acceptable. The most acceptable solutions are the ones persons discover or invent for themselves. Nurse-managers do not supply the solutions; they supply the safety and security for the search.

Five basic concepts make up a nondirective approach for counseling the problem employee:

1. Listening
2. Clarifying
3. Withholding advice
4. Minimizing authority
5. Keeping the interview issue-centered

Listening seems easy to carry out, but it is difficult for most because in listening they must not react or judge. Instead of disagreeing with or accusing the speaker, the active listener makes no judgment but instead encourages the speaker to talk. Active listening requires objectivity, respect, knowledge of self, and confidentiality. It is impossible to make someone over in another's image, so it is up to the nurse-manager to assist staff members in working out their problems at their own levels of development. Personal prejudices and biases must be recognized and then discounted. Above all, active listening holds in confidence all information that was given in confidence.

Clarifying is important because strong emotions can lead to confused thinking. Persons in the grip of a strong emotional reaction look at things subjectively and with considerable bias. The nurse-manager's role is to act as a mirror, grasp the feeling expressed, and reflect that feeling back to the individual.

Repeated clarification helps a problem employee acquire insight into the problem. The problem and the solution are the responsibility of the employee, not the nurse-manager. Recognizing the problem for exactly what it is, the employee may realize that what was a baffling and overwhelming situation can be corrected when it is examined from a different perspective.

Withholding advice keeps problem employees on the track of solving their own problems. The nurse-manager should come to the counseling session with all the available facts and then suggest to the employee that they study the facts together to determine if there is a theme or a trend. It is not the manager's concern to tell the difficult employee the course of action that the top executive thinks should be followed. As mentioned before, an employee is more apt to follow solutions that the employee has designed personally.

Minimizing authority is important in counseling because it is up to the nurse-manager to get problem employees to express their frustrations without fear of retaliation. There should be no reminder of a superior-subordinate relationship. One objective of a counseling session is to obtain relief for the frustrated employee, and this can be accomplished once the employee has been given permission to release personal hostilities and fears. With anger and fear out of the way, employees may feel better and become more inclined to see the problem as one created by themselves rather than something others have done to them.

Keeping the session issue-centered is another requirement for a counseling session. The employee's remarks must be accepted as a statement of that issue, regardless of what the employee says. The nurse-manager should accept the statements without judgment as they evolve. The objective is to understand how the employee feels and how the employee is in "pain." Conveying this acceptance is important because persons with problems are likely to feel ashamed, rejected, or different. If a person uses angry words and angry gestures, the nurse-manager should not react as if the issue were a personal one but instead should find out what is causing the anger. When the nurse-manager accepts both the individual and the emotion as important, the problem employee is helped already.

Expression of feelings makes it possible to consider the situation and other persons in a more neutral way. Until some of the electric charge has been diffused, and a state of emotional stabilizing has been established, the problem employee is not receptive, and any suggestion of change is met with resentment. To a frustrated individual a suggestion that the individual should change is regarded as an attack, and this aggravates the condition to be corrected. Punishment has a similar effect because it also makes the expression of anger difficult. Punishment increases the frustrated condition rather than correcting it. The nurse-manager must create a relationship in which expressing feelings is safe.

It is important to respond to the problem employee in an environment in which criticism is positive. The nurse-manager should pay direct attention to the employee because the employee is the most important person at that time. If some feedback is negative, the manager should handle it by giving the negative part first and the positive part last so that the latter is part of healing. The nurse-manager should talk about the immediate and tell the employee what it will be like after the problem is solved. Any comments about how the employee will reach the solution should be avoided. The idea is to take one step at a time. Concentrating on one phase of criticism makes the problem easier to deal with.

The end of the meeting should be marked by praise. It is best to close the session with a word on a positive subject without exaggeration. The nurse-manager must recognize that the manager's personal point of view is not the only way of doing things. The manager should let the employee know that the situation can be improved by working together. At the close of the meeting the employee should be invited to recount the discussion. If there are points of confusion, this is the time to define the views.

Retraining

It is up to the nurse-manager to determine the competencies that are required to provide patients with care that is satisfactory. Individualized educational programs designed to ameliorate deficiencies and sensitize employees to the job's requirements can be developed in formats to meet the determined needs.

In this realm of individualized education, mutual recognition of the deficiency and the course of self-growth action to be followed is vital. The preceptor-apprentice model is an effective method for bringing an employee up to standard. The nurse-manager acts as the preceptor with the employee in designing and guiding the upgrading process. Work groups assist the education function with full knowledge that this is being done with systematic objectives. This process is a formalization of what was previously an informal process on a hit-or-miss basis. Mutually agreed to criteria or objectives in the program should be established.

If deemed necessary, educational media can be used in the process. Programmed instruction, informal education conferences, and videos are part of the supportive process. Efforts, including individual conferences and counseling, should be documented and should include comments on employee responsiveness to education. It is helpful to the learning process to make corrections or observations tactfully "on the spot." Learning or change that occurs as a part of the work experience is helpful. Finally, the educational outcomes must be evaluated to measure the degree of change and ascertain whether a new acceptable level of performance has been reached.

Transfers

The challenge to the nurse manager lies in retaining the individual who can do the job, the individual who has the skills and attitudes necessary to perform but who is not performing satisfactorily in a specific job. The key to keeping this person for the hospital may lie in a carefully selected transfer to another unit.

A transfer can be the result of many factors. These include sublearning performance, poor matching of person to job, and dissatisfaction stemming from a plethora of employment-related environmental factors. Ineffective employee performance may be resolved by moving the employee into another environment in the hospital.

The transfer of an employee is neither punishment nor a retaliatory measure. It should be considered a management strategy with a twofold purpose. Most importantly, a transfer is an attempt to maximize utilization and productivity and to salvage an employee in whom the hospital already has a significant investment in recruitment, orientation, and educational costs.

Additionally, an employee's performance deficiencies may be caused by the work or management environment. Physical impairment, stresses at home, and personality incompatibilities can keep an employee from meeting the job expectations. The nurse-manager has little control over these factors. In such instances a transfer may salvage employees for both the hospital and themselves.

The transfer becomes a step in the "due process" of a documented process for handling subproductive employees. Transferring problem employees can be an important part of the hospital's human resource program. Wherever a transfer is to be instigated, the employee must be involved early in the process. The nurse-manager should inform the employee that a transfer is being considered. The reasons for this action should then be discussed fully and documented. The transfer should not be an abrupt change but a carefully planned event. The employee must know exactly what is happening and why.

As a supportive action the transfer should be accomplished in the same manner as any other personnel action. The entire event should be executed before the nurse-manager becomes committed to firing the employee and before the employee's anger level is beyond repair.

To determine where to transfer the problem employee, the nurse-manager must assess the employee's skills and competencies. The performance needs of the new job must be examined. The transfer must be a sincere attempt to match the needs of the hospital with the talents of the employee. Different talents should be used on the new job. A new start means a chance to use another set of professional skills. The new manager must be aware that a transfer has been made for a constructive purpose. Managers need to be aware of the value of the process both to the involved individual and to the hospital. The transfer must not be seen as rehabilitation but more as a refitting of the employee to hospital requirements.

Termination

Employees become problems because they cannot cope with conflicting choices, changes, and conditions. When problems cannot be resolved, the only answer may be termination.

Termination is perhaps one of the more difficult tasks a nurse-manager must perform. Both the manager and the employee are uncomfortable. When approached as managerial accountability and a process, termination can be handled more easily. Problem employees should understand through ongoing counseling and documentation that a point may be reached at which a determination will be made, either by the employee or the hospital, that their needs are no longer congruent. At this point a severing of the employment relationship, voluntarily or involuntarily, will take place.

As part of a process, termination must be handled in a direct, yet human, manner. The nurse-manager should not judge an individual as good or bad but should refer to documented performance evaluations and past counseling sessions. It should be pointed out that a real attempt has been made to match the individual and the organization, that a logical process has been followed, and that it has been concluded that a hospital and individual match cannot be reasonably made.

Certain humane attitudes and sensitive means can be used by the hospital to reduce the impact of terminations. These include making the action a routine, openness and candor with the employee, documentation of performance, and constructive interviews that include suggestions for future opportunities.

When confronted with unpleasant events, employees will go through stages associated with loss and grieving: denial, anger, depression, acceptance, and possible positive or constructive action.

Denial, at its most simple definition, is a rejection of the facts. It takes the form of insisting that there must be some mistake, declining to admit that anything wrong was done, or saying that the nurse-manager has made a wrong decision. Bargaining is a frequent aspect of this stage. Trying to negotiate for a few more days, a different job, a pay cut, or another chance are some examples. In some cases persons ask for reviews of records and request authentication from higher levels of management in the organization. The grievance process itself is an attempt to deal fairly with employees who feel they did not have due process.

Anger often is experienced in the death of a job. It is easy to see how some of the reactions occurring during denial lead into anger. Requests become demands, questions turn into statements of appeals, and threats become hostile actions. Productive anger is healthy, and when channeled into an activity, it can achieve a purpose.

Depression produces fatigue and despair. The targets of anger become sources of despair. The world seems to be against the terminated employee; this seems to be the worst of all possible events and the worst time for it to happen. Depression is the most destructive stage because it feeds upon itself and is difficult to end. Depression "proves" that the person should be depressed. Depression permits and encourages lethargy and inaction while providing scapegoats and allowing excuses to be acceptable.

Accepting the reality of the termination and then accepting that the employee is the only one who can provide action will put the employee on the road to healing.

Dealing with Defensiveness

All positions in nursing management deal with the defensive employee. When caught by the verbal backlash of the angry physician, the dissatisfied patient, or the frustrated staff member, physiology reverts to a fight-or-flight mechanism. Defensiveness is a coping reaction to a perceived or real attack between the self and others.

Defensive reactions are caused by an attempt to protect either a personal or a public image or by a perceived invasion of personal turf and territory. Directly or indirectly, the message has been received that a personal power base is vulnerable to invasion.

Defensive behavior also comes from an elevated anxiety level because of guilt, blame, and shame caused by not living up to expectations that others hold for a person's achievement.

Defensive employees set up a psychologic fence around their egos and their physical territories. Defensiveness is a protective rather than a projective type of coping. When another person has difficulty comprehending the consequences of proposed change or lack of control, defensiveness can be expected. When there is suspicion that rights and judgments are being infringed upon, defensive behavior can be anticipated.

If a disgruntled staff nurse comes charging into the nurse-manager's office, the manager's first reaction is protective. Because the staff nurse is ready to charge, it is difficult to remain other-person focused. When the nurse-manager is on the receiving end of defensiveness and anger, the focus of words and questions must be kept on the other person. It takes practice and patience to develop nonjudgmental listening. (even though the speaker is behaving immaturely).

If the defensive person asks a lot of questions in the first part of the encounter, it is important for the nurse-manager to restrict answers and begin to ask questions because it is important to discover who owns the problem. The defensive person might be doing management a personal service by bringing attention to a problem that management was not aware of.

Three interactions produce defensive behavior: hinderance, helplessness, and hopelessness. Staff members who feel they look inferior, inadequate, or incompetent cause ripples of unrest. Any conflicts or changes in the working relationship can leave employees feeling susceptible to blocks and interferences. Fearing these interferences, the defensive person will engage in justification as a means of self-protection.

Defensive behavior seldom occurs unless a change is perceived. Change represents an attack on self-vested interests. Defensiveness is a nonconstructive reaction to a real or rumored change. It also can occur after looking and listening for the hidden agenda of what the other person did not say. Defensive employees feel that they are being manipulated or that they are not being informed of what is really going on. Personal and professional practice expectations that are not being met also can cause defensiveness.

Staff nurses who feel hindered in their performance while attempting to gain recognition and respect also can feel helpless. They both hear and generate rumors based on supposition. When they feel they no longer have control over the direction of the administration of their duties, they suffer intense pangs of hopelessness. The consequences of this hopelessness develop into defensiveness.

Behaviors do not change until emotions are dissipated. In confronting the angry employee, the nurse-manager should separate the employee from the rest of the staff and let the employee rant and rave. If the nurse-manager absorbs the anger without becoming defensive, the emotion will dissipate. It is a wise move *not* to give answers or solutions but to suggest how to generate alternative ways to solve the problem. Winning with defensive employees does not include giving them advice. Defensive persons look for relationships.

As a strategy to dissolve defensiveness, troubled persons

should be assisted in trying to find alternative solutions to their problems. They also need understanding and appreciation for their position. Even though persons who are angry and defensive are difficult to listen to, they should be allowed to talk at least 85% of the time. The manager should allow them to verbalize and then focus on identifying the actual problem, the cause of deviation, and the differences in position. Often it is the deviation that is increasing the defensiveness.

Defensive employees want feedback in a one-to-one encounter to satisfy their needs. A critical point before the employee leaves the confrontation is to take time to renegotiate how a problem can be handled in the future if a difference of opinion should occur. This is the time to decide how to deal with potential differences. Opening the lines for future problem solving can reassure and secure an interpersonal contract for ongoing working relationships.

By now nurse-managers should be aware that individuals use defensive behavior as a coping technique, an abutment, against the pains of rejection by others. Here is the summary of the four steps nurse-managers can use to deal with defensiveness:

1. *Active listening.* The manager should listen actively to what the other person is saying and ask questions to ensure clarity of understanding. The other person should be allowed to talk and emotionally unwind until completely finished.
2. *Feedback.* The manager should feed back what the manager has heard the other person say. If there is any misunderstanding, the other person can correct the manager's interpretation. The manager should let defensive persons see that the manager cares and trusts them enough to allow them to be human and even make mistakes. The manager should be willing to work with the employee and be grateful for the opportunity to improve staff relations.
3. *Waiting.* Nurse-managers should wait until the emo-

tions have been dissipated and then share with the individual their points of view of the problem. They should not accuse or intimate any "wrong." This is not the time to give advice, but it is the time to share thoughts as objectively and factually as possible.
4. *Recalling.* When the confrontation is over, the manager should ask the other person to recall what has transpired. If there are any points of confusion or misunderstanding, the issues should be carefully redefined.

When defensive staff nurses trample on a nurse-manager's ego or assault the manager's power base, a nurse-manager who cares about the staff nurses will ask questions, especially about the staff members' personal selves. When staff nurses begin to tell the nurse-manager who they really are, they may discover that together management and staff can work together in mutual understanding and trust as new patterns for management develop.

Chapter 9

The Emerging Patterns of Management

The previous chapters have alerted nurse-managers to ways to meet crises in health care, define an accurate perception of events, and develop management skills. Now it is necessary to step back and look at the bigger picture.

Slowly but surely the health care industry is undergoing deep-rooted changes. This difficult time of transformation for hospitals must be considered from a broad view of social and economic history.

The course of human development has seen at least two instances of revolutionary change: the change from a hunting and gathering society to an agricultural one and the change from an agrarian society to an industrial one.

The Changing World of Health Care

The industrial society changed an essentially self-sufficient, health-satisfied person into one who was almost totally dependent on the services of the physician. As mass production of health required the standardization of procedures, new communities were formed and housed in the cement and steel structures of the hospital. The new instruments and measurements invented and tooled to satisfy the physician-expert required specialization by the nurse. Healing came to be seen as a product provided by the physician and nurse in a health delivery bureaucracy. Healing was "produced" by the physicians and nurses within a hospital and "consumed" by the patient.

As the hospitals grew, they became healing factories in which hundreds of laborers were drawn together under a single roof to concentrate on energy, a consumer population, and a work force. These healing factories burgeoned into one of the biggest industries in the Unites States, possibly because maximizing was considered economical or because "big" had become synonymous with "better." As the industrialization of healing spread, the high cost of instrumentation and the specialization of the labor force required synchronization. Time and technology became related to money.

Unfortunately, high technology meant high cost. This high cost for individual patient care brought about yet another industry dependent on a large number of well participants whose chances for illness were low. It was in this way that the health insurance industry became an offshoot of the health care industry.

When state and federal governments started meeting the health needs of the elderly, a different consumer population came to the front. Here was a group whose chances of illness were high. These payment-for-service businesses watched as profit-and-loss statements wavered in precarious balance. Something drastic had to be done. Hospitalizations became limited to the acute phase of illness. Insurance payments were made according to DRGs. A new interpretation of the hospital mission emerged. Hospitals no longer could give service without consideration of cost. As a result, nursing too had to be considered not only as a mission of caring but also as a business of service that could look at the economics of healing.

To run the healing business, ideas of scientific management emphasizing centralization of information and chains of command were instigated by many hospital administrators. Judging from the actions of administrators who operated under these ideas, a common value system developed. The scientific manager believed the following: big is better, low costs win, analysis forecasts, no one disagrees with management, all decisions come from the top, power is for dominance, money is a motivator, inspection controls quality, persons must be kept in alignment, and, finally, growth guarantees success.

This value system supported an industrial society in the early part of the 20th century in which the labor force was largely informally educated and less skilled, with high turnover and high conflict. There was a clear distinction between nurses and supervisors. Nursing tasks were quite straightforward: massage, tepid baths, poultices, mustard plasters, 24-hour soaks, special diets, immobilization, and complete bed rest. Nursing supervisors within the health care setting were, in the industrial tradition, directors of their organizations. They set goals, made policies, implemented practices, and measured results. Their job was to rule their subordinates.

Contrast this with the emerging design of health care organizations. Today nurses must be formally educated, sophisticated employees who have learned complex, intellectual tasks. They have become experts in administering chemicals to alter disease states, in applying and reading electronic instrumentation, in assisting in the intrusive procedures of diagnosis, and in helping in surgical procedures of reconstruction. Nurses also have become engaged in creating, processing, and distributing the health information that is the strategic resource of the new health delivery system.

As in all other professional work, it is becoming necessary to view a nurse's individual knowledge as an economic value. This signals a new era, in an era of transformation in which circumstances necessitate a major shift in ideas. Thomas Kuhn,[1] the historian of science, has pointed out that major changes take place only occasionally in what he calls "paradigm shifts." These are the times when the ways people do things become so inappropriate that they cannot be used and must be replaced by more appropriate ways. This idea fits the changing world of the hospital as it moves from an industrial society to an informational one. It is time to transform old thinking into new patterns for more appropriate endeavors. This marks the paradigm shift.

The Paradigm Shift

A paradigm is a pattern of thought, a scheme for understanding and explaining certain aspects of reality. A paradigm shift is a new way of thinking about old problems. For example, since the early 1900s leading management thinkers assumed that Taylor's industrial paradigm,[2,3] his description of time related to product and profit, could be used to interpret everything in terms of the advantages of division of labor. It would explain the merits of a hierarchical organization and the advantages of an industrial society.

However, as behavioral scientists worked toward the elusive answers about a worker's motivation, bits of data refused to fit into Taylor's scheme of things. This is typical of any paradigm. Eventually, too many puzzles emerge outside the old framework and put a strain on it. At this point of crisis, someone had a unique idea. New insight explained the apparent contradictions, and a new perspective was introduced. The new principle forced a more comprehensive theory that made the revolutionary idea not destructive but instructive.

Just as the discovery of hormones, antibiotics, antihistamines, and psychotropic drugs gave evidence of a revolutionary idea in the health delivery industry, so the Hawthorne Experiments[4] gave clues of the new paradigm for the business management industry. These experiments resolved many riddles about scientific management. Workers wanted tangible evidence of social importance: acceptance as members of a group, recognition of their useful skills, and acknowledgment of their specialized technologic information. The old mechanical rules of industry (time and motion) had become insufficient explanations of increased productivity under adverse conditions. Understanding of the work forces had shifted from one paradigm to another.

According to Naisbitt,[5] other social and economic events give evidence of a larger paradigm shift from the industrial to the information paradigm:

1. In today's organizations, the overwhelming majority of service workers are actually engaged in creating, processing, and distributing information.
2. A highly personal value system has evolved to compensate for the impersonal nature of technology.
3. The nature of electronic money transactions has shifted the United States from being a self-sufficient national economy to being part of an interdependent global economy.
4. The use of computer programs to project trends and futures has shifted business management from short-term profits to long-term planning.
5. There is a moving away from centralization: In politics government is being transferred to state and local levels. In business the focus is on local rather than national demands. In culture ethnic diversity is recognized rather than the melting pot idea.
6. Americans have moved away from the institutions of medicine, business, and schools and are learning to help themselves in matters of health, employment, and education.
7. The ethic of participation has changed—people expect to be a part of the process of decision making.
8. Large conglomerates are being reconstructed into smaller units.
9. Population has shifted from the high industrial states of Michigan, Massachusetts, Ohio, and New York to the high technology states of Texas, New Mexico, Arizona, and California.
10. Persons in today's world are individualistic and expect a wide range of choices.

These are patterns (trends) that confirm a larger shift.

Implications of this larger shift involve a principle that was present all along but not noticed by managers. It includes the old as a partial truth while allowing for things to work out in other ways as well. The perspective of the new paradigm transforms traditional knowledge and new observations and reconciles their apparent contradictions.

This new pattern of thought about the use of an individual's information and ability does more than the old industrial notion. It can predict the process of individual motivation for goal attainment more accurately. It sheds light on new research.

With all its advantages this new pattern might be expected to catch hold rather quickly, but that has not happened. The problem is that managers cannot embrace the new paradigm unless they let go of the old ideas about scientific management. It is a change that cannot come about gradually. "Like the gestalt switch," Kuhn[1] said, "it must occur all at once." The new paradigm is not figured out but suddenly seen.

A new paradigm nearly always is received with either coolness or hostility. Social importance, self-actualization, need for achievement, and release of motivation are ideas that seem to contradict the tried and true methods for tying profits to an economic use of people-time. These ideas were met with coolness. To the scientific manager they appeared bizarre because without examining the hard data of time, motion, and production, behavioral scientists had made an intuitive leap. They predicted that satisfying a person's internal drive could enhance company profits.

This new perspective centers on the importance of the individual's needs and know-how and demands a switch. Now the power of the new paradigm to accomplish corporate goals is being recognized. The paradigm shift, a reconceptualization of the structure, responsibilities, and goals of an organization, will take place in response to five pressures.

Pressures that Affect the Paradigm Shift

According to Toffler,[6] the new wave of thinking, the paradigm shift, will be precipitated by five critical changes in the actual conditions of production:

1. Changes in the physical environment
2. Changes in the social environment
3. Changes in the role of information
4. Changes in government and organization
5. Changes in morality

These changes are forcing the health delivery system into a multifaceted, multipurposeful shape.

In the health care system the first of these pressures, the physical environment, springs from medical technology. New medical miracles such as organ transplantation, artificial joints, and artificial kidneys require special equipment such as telemetry, orthopedic appliances, and dialysis machines. These and other similar technologic demands require special care units within the hospital and cost millions of dollars. New developments in medical technology compel health care to be one of the largest industries in the United States; medical costs rank in the top percentage of the GNP.

Measured in any way, demands on the health care industry will continue to escalate. As a result hospitals will send alarm signals: shortened hospital stays, closing of obstetric units, and admittance determined by ability to pay. In addition, increasingly more warnings will signify that health care no longer can be organized as it was in the past.

The second pressure springs from a change in the social environment in which the hospital finds itself. The hospital is far more organized than before. At one time each hospital department operated independently. Now there must be daily interaction between physicians, nurses, physical and occupational therapists, pharmacists and so forth. These professionals are being forced to act as a health team on each patient-care unit.

In this densely crowded social environment, every hospital action has repercussive impacts not only on the individual worker but also on organized groups represented by professional associations and trade unions. Decisions that affect the health worker's education, employment, or upward mobility put a far greater responsibility than ever before on the hospital for its social process as well as its economic service.

A third set of pressures reflects the sphere of information. Today far more information is exchanged between health workers and patients. To maintain an equilibrium between illness and wellness, information has become central to patient-care service. A new dimension has emerged in regard to patient-care education. Now the hospital is seen as producer of health information for wellness as well as a producer of a healing service for illness recovery.

A fourth pressure on the health care system arises from the political scene. The rapid decentralization of government and the acceleration of technologic change are reflected in a tremendously complex government. Both state and federal governments designate special agencies to oversee the health care of their constituents, protect the working public from industrial accidents, provide for a safe environment, safeguard hazardous storage of nuclear and chemical wastes, and preserve the quality of food and drugs. These agencies, each with its own priorities, are poorly coordinated and are in a perpetual turmoil of reorganization. Whether it is care of the average citizen, the unwed mother, the victim of an industrial accident, the senior citizen, the undocumented worker, or the poor, every hospital finds itself increasingly ensnarled in political restraints regardless of whether it is on the local, state, or national level.

Finally, as the industrial pattern of thought declines, and its value system shatters, the fifth pressure placed on hospital organization becomes apparent: moral pressure. Management behavior once accepted as normal is reinterpreted as degrading and disrespectful. The members of the organization must be managed in other ways than by cajoling, directing, ruling, limiting, and ordering.

The new information paradigm places a premium on managing the development of human resources. Greater attention is given to an individual's technologic information for the hospital's mission, a person's role expectations, the person's contribution to a specific philosophy, and the fit of personal and organizational values as deemed by the hospital culture.

The hospital culture has a powerful impact on the morale and productivity of nurses and other health care workers. Those associated with the hospital can either accept or reject its culture.

The Importance of Hospital Culture

Culture is an invisible web that holds a group of persons together in a unique life-style.[7] Silently, attitudes and rules are interwoven into social interactions as a way of adapting to the environment.

As has been inferred in chapter 2, a hospital culture is multidimensional. It encompasses a body of ideas and concepts, customs and traditions, and procedures and habits for coping in its own particular environment. A hospital culture weaves a web of subsystems into a strong wash-and-wear fabric that can be used to weather the storm in adapting and understanding. It is the interweaving process that helps personnel achieve hospital objectives and preserve the hospital's values.

The hospital depends on nurse-managers to weave nurse energy and information and transform them into patient care that reflects policies and procedures, attitudes and principles, and ethics and values determined by the hospital culture. What must be recognized is that management practices are in transition as a new hospital culture emerges and the old culture declines.

Declining and Emerging Patterns of Management

There are two patterns of hospital management: the disappearing industrial-age model and the emerging information-age model (Table 9-1).

Culture Component	Industrial Model	Information Model
Metaphor	Factory	Corporation
Structure	Hierarchy	Matrix
Role learning	Defined by task	Defined by talent
Patient-care business	Routine nurse operations	Specializations
Power	Concentrated at top	Dispersed to team
Communication	Vertical, top down	Horizontal, lateral sharing
Health mission	Confined to hospitalized patient	Expanded to teaching prevention and home care
Nurse education	Depends on community colleges and universities for basic nurse education	Expects business theory for nurse managers, learning theory for staff and patient education, and physiology psychosociology for patient care specializations
Recreation	An after-hours activity	Part of the work hard—play hard ethic within the organization

Table 9-1—Comparison of Management Models

They can be recognized in places where nurses are paid for the "sweat of their brow" or in places where nurses are paid for their "technologic know-how." The differences become more evident when each type of management is examined.

The disappearing industrial model for hospital administration molded by Taylor[2,3] his description of time proclaims the need for scientific management that can relate time to money and bureaucracy to efficiency. The metaphor that most aptly describes this model is the factory system whose structure is hierarchal. Here role learning is defined by task and functions that can be described as static and predictable. Patient-care business is managed by routine nurse operations. Power of nursing administration is concentrated at the top for decision making to dominate the lower echelon: the staff nurses and nurses' aides. Communication is delivered by a vertical path from the top down. Motivation is expected when monetary reward is given for achievement. The health mission depends on patients who are hospitalized for diagnosis, medical control, surgical procedures, and complete recovery. Formal nurse education depends on the community colleges and universities for basic patient care. (The business of hospital economics is part of informal role learning.) Recreation is considered an after-hours activity.

The emerging information model for nursing management is influenced by the theorists McGregor[8] and Maslow.[9] They stressed the need for development of human resources that can release an individual's motivation, a situation that will lead to attainment of matched personal and organizational goals. The metaphor that most aptly describes this model is a corporate culture that has a matrix structure. Here role learning is defined by talent and functions that can be described as dynamic and adaptable. Hospital business is managed by mobile personnel of different specializations who are always ready for change and continuous reorganization. Hospital management power is dispersed to the health delivery team for group decision making. Communication follows a horizontal path, and ideas are shared laterally. Motivation is released when the team members are given the opportunity for and recognition of personal and professional development. The health mission adds new concepts of health teaching for prevention and at-home care for healing during the recovery phase of illness. Formal education is recommended for promotional consideration (eg, business education for managers, learning theory for nurse and patient education, and biopsychosocial sciences for patient-care specialists). Recreation is a part of the work hard/play hard ethic within the hospital organization.

Managers of the New Paradigm

As these culture components become entwined in an economically successful hospital oriented toward technical information, the essential functions of management that focus on the development of human resources emerge. According to Levitt,[10] management consists of the rational assessment of a situation and the systematic selection of goals and purpose: the systematic development of strategies to achieve these goals; the marshalling of the required resources; the rational design, organization, direction, and control of the activities required to attain the selected purposes; and, finally, the motivating and rewarding of persons to do the work. In other words, the manager is the problem-solver who adapts impersonal attitudes toward goals that are deeply embedded in the culture of the organization. Managers tend to view work as an enabling process involving combinations of persons and ideas interacting to establish strategies and make decisions.

Furthermore, managers for the new paradigm, as Zaleznik[11] defined them, help the process along by a range of skills, including calculating the interests in opposition, staging and timing the surfacing of controversial issues, and reducing tensions. In this enabling process, managers use tactics flexibly. They negotiate and bargain on the one hand and use rewards and delegate power on the other.

Re-emphasizing Burns,[12] this is a reciprocal process of mobilizing persons with certain motives, values, and economic and educational resources in a context of competition and conflict to realize goals held independently or mutually by both leaders and followers.

One way of assessing the reciprocal manager style is to examine four critical functions of management: leadership, motivation, communication, and use of power.

Leadership is a function of management, not a specific role. It involves the activities of persuasion, invitation, argument, affectionate devotion, and the provision of problem situations for learning group decision making. Leadership function is an interpersonal influence that is directed through communication and exercised in situations to attain an organization's specific goals. Internal forces that influence leadership are the value system, trust in others, and a need for credibility. External forces that shape leadership are the subordinates' interest in the job, individual needs for self-support, the workers' abilities to acquire new knowledge, the employees' willingness to assume responsibility, and readiness for decision making. Situational forces that affect behavior of leaders are the type of organization, the culture of the work group, and the kind of work to be accomplished. Two aspects of leadership function are interrelated: the efficient and wise exercise of power and the presentation of a vision that can express a common goal within a shared value system. As power and vision interact, a relationship of mutual stimulation develops. The leader recognizes the self-distinction need of the follower and seeks to satisfy that need while the follower recognizes the vision of the leader as a way to accomplish self-distinction and is motivated to attain the organization's goal.

Thus, a major function of nurse-managers is to shape values that help define the direction of the hospital and allow an orderly determination of individual goals, options, and priorities. Many nurse-managers will be threatened by this concept of leadership because it involves the loss of formal authority.

The first step that any hospital's management group should take is to consciously define the institution's values.[13] Some examples include participation, responsibility, personal growth, competence, equity, effectiveness, integrity, respect, accountability, and creativity.

The next task should be to design a goal statement for each of these values. The aforementioned list of values generates these goal statements shown in Table 9-2.

Value	Goal
Participation	To encourage maximum participation in the total health care process
Responsibility	To give staff members as much responsibility as they can handle with patients or employees
Personal growth	To anticipate a continued individual effort for personal growth
Competence	To create an environmental demand for competence
Equity	To encourage equity and fairness in all hospital transactions
Effectiveness	To promote effectiveness by maximizing resources
Integrity	To create an environment that expects personal integrity and honesty
Respect	To foster an environment for mutual concern and respect of the individual's personhood
Accountability	To expect accountability from each member as well as the total organization
Creativity	To foster creativity and innovative ideas

Table 9-2—Hospital Values Related to Hospital Goals

To shape these hospital values into individual goals, the nurse-manager must shift from a hierarchal relationship with staff nurses and patient service employees to a more collaborative, collegial relationship.

Leadership, as a reciprocal process, will demand that nurse-managers spend more time socializing and teaching the hospital's values. If one of the hospital's values is effective patient care, specific examples must be provided to staff members in terms of their own work to match their own goals to goals of the hospital.

When personal growth is a value of the hospital, nurse-managers will need to spend more time training and retraining workers. This will include not only technical skills but also interpersonal skills of listening, communicating, and problem solving.

When participation is a value, the nurse-manager will have to highlight the interdependence of work units such as the pharmacy, radiology, laboratory, and nursing services.

When creativity is a value, the nurse-manager will have to make greater use of personal attention for innovation as a reward.

When accountability is a value, the nurse-manager will have to give greater attention to better ways of providing performance feedback. Specifically, staff members must see how their behavior reflects job responsibility.

In the large part, reciprocal leadership implies that there is another function of management that requires a clear understanding of motivation.

Motivation refers to an individual's goal-directed behavior that is characterized by the process of selecting and directing certain personal actions among voluntary activities to achieve goals.[14] It is influenced not only by an individual's characteristic needs, interests, attitudes, and goals but also by organizational tasks, managerial practices, and organizational climate. Motivation is not generated externally; it comes from within the individual. It energizes, directs, and sustains individual work behavior that is a result of interaction between the individual and the environmental factors. According to Herzberg,[15] the factors involved in producing motivation (job satisfaction) are found in job content. They are the stimuli for personal growth, are intrinsic to the job, and include achievement opportunities, recognition of achievement, the work itself, responsibility, and personal advancement or distinction.

In primary nursing when a nurse is asked to provide the complete care for a group of patients, the motivators involved will be responsibility, achievement, and recognition.

Granting additional authority to staff nurses for making

decisions about dress codes, shift time, and assignments will involve the motivators of responsibility, achievement, and recognition.

Assigning the achieving nurses specific or specialized tasks, enabling them to become experts, involves the motivators of responsibility, growth, and advancement.

In other words, motivation requires that the nurse-manager match patient-care tasks and hospital routines with the staff nurses' expectations for personal growth, achievement, and recognition. Motivation is a continuous management function and calls for open communication between managers and staff members.

As previously pointed out, communication is the essence of organized activity and depends on the quality and availability of information. Usually an organizational system of communication is created by setting up formal systems of responsibilities and delegating explicit duties. However, research has shown that groups tend to depart from formal statements to create other channels of communication.[16] In other words, informal systems of communication emerge.

The "excellent companies" studied by Peters and Waterman[16] had vast networks of informal, open communication. This type of communication is a process of exchanging information between individuals across organizational boundaries without concern for hierarchal office. It is face-to-face information shared in "real time"—the moment an issue comes up. (For further information about empowerment through open communication, see Kanter.[17]) The patterns and intensity of open communication put the right people into contact with each other regularly. The regularity of contact and opportunities for peer competition keep the chaotic, hierarchal properties of an organization under control.

Open communication stresses access across segments through an open door. Open-door policies mean that employees at all levels have access, theoretically, to anyone to ask questions and to criticize. In other words, members of the organization talk to each other a lot without a lot of paper work or formal routine.

The excellent companies had five attributes of open communication that encouraged creativity and innovation:[16]

1. *Open communication was informal.* There were endless, unscheduled meetings. Persons from different departments casually gathered together to discuss problems. This ensured that the right persons were in touch with one another regularly.

2. *Open communication was intense.* Whenever senior managers made a presentation, everyone became involved with a free flow of questions. Employees did not hesitate to say what they wanted to say or to question their superiors. There was an open, confrontation-oriented management style in which all individuals went after the issues bluntly and straightforwardly.

3. *Open communication was physically close.* The most productive companies were located in campuslike settings where persons were placed close to one another to increase the probability of communication. Blackboards were found everywhere to encourage immediate and graphic exchange of ideas.

4. *Open communication was used as a forcing device.* Excellent companies encouraged free thinkers and gave them the status of the elite. They were given free rein to experiment, question across lines, and gather all the information that could bring about change. Their job was to shake up the system and to force innovation into the organization.

5. *Open communication held tight control.* When communication had few boundaries, more people had control. Whenever money was spent, there was genuine interest because many people checked up informally to see how things were going. Not only managers but also peers held the power of influence.

Nurse-managers of the new paradigm probably will find the concept of open communication most difficult. In hospitals clinging to the industrial tradition, communication can be described in characteristics that are the opposites of open communication:

1. *Formal communication is rigid.* Status symbols and boundary limits that demonstrate rigid communication are everywhere. Physicians eat in private dining rooms. Supervisors dress differently and wear laboratory coats over their street clothes. Staff nurses cling to white as part of their uniform—colored tops perhaps, but always white pants and shoes. Volunteers can be recognized by their pastel smocks. Uniforms for respiratory therapists and janitors are also color coded. Messages are sent by physicians' orders, the "day" book, memos from the directors, and rules and regulations from standard procedures.

2. *Formal communication is tempered.* Suggestions to supervisors from staff nurses are guided through "proper" channels in which the individual's innovative ideas are buffered from personal criticism.

3. *Formal communication channels are physically distant.* Whether it is hospital business, student nurse education, or continuing education for staff nurses, managers and educators are housed in off-unit offices or off-site campuses.

4. *Formal communication is used as a status quo device.* Verbal and nonverbal messages about ethics and values remind hospital personnel not to disturb the existing state of affairs. Rocking the boat is not accepted. The old tried and true ways must be maintained.

5. *Formal communication provides an escape from individual recognition and responsibility.* It is not unusual for a nurse to withhold ideas about money savings or improved care. Past experiences have shown there is no

opportunity for self-distinction. Too many staff nurses have discovered that as their suggestions ascended the steps of the hierarchy, so many others were involved that the name of the innovator, the person responsible for the suggestion, was lost.

In summary, formal communication is rigid, tempered, physically distant, maintaining, and lacks opportunities for self-distinction. Open communication is informal, intense, physically close, change expecting, and peer controlling. Even though open communication may mean that problems as well as successes cannot be kept secret, it is an important function of managing in the new paradigm. Information and ideas must flow freely. Technical data and alternative points of view must be gathered easily. It is communication based on debate among peers, rather than information transmission based on top-down authority, that determines the control system and the use of power.

The Changing Intensity of Power Bases

According to French and Raven,[18] the phenomena of power and influence involve a dyadic relation between two individuals. The focus on the follower (the subordinate) upon whom power is exerted defines the bases of power and explains the interactions of social influence.

As previously discussed, there are several bases of power, but five important types are reward, coercive, legitimate, referent, and expert.

In a management perspective reward power depends on the nurse-manager's ability to administer positive experiences and decrease negative experiences. For instance, when a nurse-manager gives a staff nurse the opportunity for self-direction and creative expression, the result will be reward power for the nurse-manager.

The strength of coercive power depends on the perceived magnitude of a punishment experience. Just as a personal responsibility can serve as a basis for reward power, the ability to withhold personal responsibility will be perceived as coercive power.

One basis for legitimate power is acceptance of the organizational structure. If staff members accept as right the hierarchal structure of the hospital, they will accept the legitimate authority of the nurse-manager who occupies a superior office in the hierarchy.

Referent power is based on the identification of an individual with another person. Nurse-managers should be acutely aware of the staff nurses whose bedside manner, expressed beliefs about patient care, and perceived expectations of physician-nurse interactions are similar to their own. The stronger the identification of the staff with the nurse-manager, the greater is the manager's referent power.

Expert power is based on an individual's ideas about another person's knowledge. In the management sense, the subordinate evaluates the manager's expertness in relation to personal knowledge as well as against an absolute standard. This expert power is limited to the specific areas of demonstrated knowledge.

Whether it is reward, coercive, legitimate, referent, or expert power, tomorrow's nurse-managers must recognize their own empowerment skills. The new pattern of management that is emerging in the informational age recognizes that increased technical knowledge is embedded in tasks. This means that nurse-managers cannot simply concentrate on getting the work done because they are often less knowledgeable about the work process than their subordinates. In other words, authority is centralized, but ability is inherently decentralized because it comes from practice and training rather than from definition. Although nurse-managers retain full rights to make all decisions, they have less and less ability to do so because of the advance in science and technology. Thus, even though tomorrow's nurse-managers will have legitimate power, they will have less expert power. With emphasis on the reciprocal process of management, they must develop a new strength in reward and referent power.

Tomorrow's Nurse-Manager: A Pattern for Excellence

This discussion of the broad view of social and economic events makes two facts clear: First, as a part of a larger paradigm shift, there is evidence of a declining industrial hospital model and an emerging informational hospital model. Second, these changes will affect manager function. Meeting these changes will require that tomorrow's nurse-managers develop a different pattern. It will be necessary for them to do the following:

1. *Be aware of a new value system.* Ideas of informational management that uses decentralization of information and command will be instigated by many hospital administrators. Nurse-managers who operate under these ideas will develop a common value system. They will believe that effectiveness is best, power is for delegation, self-distinction rather than money is the best motivator, management should be challenged, communication is based on peer debate rather than on top-down authority, decision making and goal setting are shared between manager and subordinate, and it is the nurse-manager who matches vision with the staff members' values and guarantees success of the hospital mission.

2. *Develop followership.* Followership is the art of guiding and enticing a group of persons to accomplish a goal. It requires an interrelationship between the wise use of power and the presentation of a vision that can be expressed through a shared value system. As vision and

values are matched, mutual stimulation occurs. It is a reciprocal process. Recognizing the self-distinction need of the follower, the guide will satisfy that need. Recognizing the vision of the guide as a way of accomplishing self-distinction, the follower will be motivated to attain the specified goal. Thus, when vision and value are matched, staff members will be motivated, and nurse-managers will attain goals.

3. *Define the motivators.* As a continuous management function, motivation must be released to energize, direct, and sustain the staff members' work behavior. It is up to the nurse-manager to define the motivating factors within the job content that stimulate staff members for personal growth. Nurse-managers need to determine staff members' perceived expectations for opportunities to achieve, to be recognized, and to be responsible.

4. *Identify the dissatisfiers.* There is a healthy side to work: a balance between the job culture and job content. When the individual employee is not in sync with hospital culture, dissatisfaction exists. The nurse-manager must identify the dissatisfiers by investigating any dissonance between staff members and company policy, administration, supervision, interpersonal relationships, working conditions, salary, status, and security.

5. *Initiate open communication.* Even though open communication may be perceived as a threat by some members of management, it is an important function of the new pattern for managing. As information and ideas flow freely, a stronger base of referent power develops. As technical data is shared, a stronger base of expert power develops. As individuals are rewarded for transmitting information, a stronger base of reward power develops. Actually, when communication has fewer boundaries, not only nurse-managers but also staff members will share in the control of health care delivery.

6. *Recognize empowerment skills.* Empowerment is an investment of authority in a subordinate so that individual can satisfy the need for self-distinction by self-direction and, at the same time, accomplish an organizational goal. It enables an individual to have the means or opportunity to accomplish a prescribed change by releasing personal energy. It is accomplished by giving the subordinate the power to act on behalf of the personal self as well as the organization. Furthermore, empowerment will be accomplished when the manager tries to do the following:

- Accept the blame for failure or mistakes.
- Share all relevant information.
- Avoid using legitimate authority by never showing impatience with progress.
- Be generous in giving credit to others for successful results.
- Encourage each individual to express personal ideas.
- State personal contributions in forms of questions.
- Refrain from imposing personal decisions.
- Encourage critical evaluation.

In this way empowerment increases the ability to get things done. Persons work better when they are doing what they like to do and are good at. Enthusiastic commitment flows out of challenge, a chance to contribute, and an opportunity to be recognized. Everyone benefits when individual needs are aligned with organizational goals. Individuals can make a difference, but they need tools and the opportunity to use them. They need to work in settings in which they are valued and supported, in which their intelli-gence and technologic information are given an opportunity to develop. They need to have personal power to initiate change.

New values, followership, motivators, identified dissatisfiers, open communication, and empowerment must be a part of the new management pattern. In anticipation of change, each nurse-manager must learn to adapt this pattern, apply it carefully, and then make sure the adaptation takes hold.

As the old hospital model declines and the new hospital model emerges, a new pattern of management that expresses an ethic of self-development is required. Individuals, not organizations, create excellence. With their unique technologic information and skill, co-workers will guide others toward excellence. Future nurse-managers will make sure that they are personally groomed for strategic thinking and have a flair for building a strong culture. Above all, tomorrow's nurse-manager must be ready with the courage to abandon the traditional.

References

1. Kuhn TS: *The Structure of Scientific Revolution*, ed 2. Chicago, University of Chicago Press, 1970.
2. Taylor FW: The principles of scientific management. *Bull Taylor Soc*, December 1916.
3. Mankin D, Ames RE Jr, Grodsky MA (eds): *Classics of Industrial and Organizational Psychology*. Oak Park, Ill, Moore Publishing Co Inc, 1980, pp 15-28.
4. Roethlisberger FJ: The Hawthorne experiments, in Natemeyer WE (ed): *Classics of Organizational Behavior*. Oak Park, Ill, Moore Publishing Co, 1978, pp 2-12.
5. Naisbitt J: *Megatrends*. New York, Warner Books Inc, 1982.
6. Toffler A: *The Third Wave*. New York, Bantam Books Inc, 1981.
7. Harris P, Moran R: *Managing Cultural Differences*. Houston, Gulf Publishing Co, 1981.
8. McGregor DM: The human side of enterprise. *Management Rev*, November 1957, pp 22-28, 88-92.
9. Maslow AH: A theory of human motivation. *Psychol Rev* 1943;50:370-396.
10. Levitt T: Management and the postindustrial society. *The Public Interest*, Summer 1975.
11. Zaleznik A: Managers and leaders: Are they different? *Harvard Bus Rev*, May/June 1977, pp 67-78.
12. Burns JM: *Leadership*. New York, Harper & Row Publishers Inc, 1978.
13. Ouchi WG: *Theory Z*. New York, Avon Books, 1981.
14. Drucker P: *Managing in Turbulent Times*. New York, Harper & Row Publishers Inc, 1980.
15. Herzberg F: One more time: How do you motivate employees? *Harvard Bus Rev*, January/February 1968, pp 58-69.
16. Peters TJ, Waterman RH: *In Search of Excellence*. New

York, Warner Books Inc, 1982.

17. Kanter RM: *The Change Masters*. New York, Simon & Schuster Inc, 1983.

18. French JRP, Raven B: The bases of social power, in Cartwright D (ed): *Studies in Social Power*. Ann Arbor, Institute for Social Research, University of Michigan, 1959, pp 150-165.

Index